MW01063787

Praise for *Lost in My Mind*

"This peek into the real-life trials and triumphs of a young woman, who survives a horrific car crash and struggles to regain academic excellence and meaningful social relationships, is a worthwhile read for anyone who needs information, inspiration, or escape from the isolation so common after traumatic brain injury."

Susan H. Connors, President/CEO,
Brain Injury Association of America

"Kelly Bouldin Darmofal showed me a world I had never experienced. Knowing the challenges, the strengths, and the perspectives that students with TBI bring to learning, I can be a better teacher for them. I admire what Kelly has accomplished in her life and her book. Anyone who cares about teaching and learning must read this remarkable story."

Louann Reid, Professor and Chair, Department of English,
Colorado State University, and former editor of *English Journal*

"*Lost in My Mind* is an exceptional, heart-rending account of one young woman's life suddenly transformed into a nightmare, and how she overcame it... a bright, happy girl who, in one night, sustains a Traumatic Brain Injury (TBI) from a car accident, changing her life forever. Kelly Darmofal's book is a triumphant example of how the human spirit can overcome life's most serious challenges."

Karen Ackerson, Executive Director of the Writer's Workshop of
Asheville, NC, and founder of the Renbourne Literary Agency

"I will never forget the day I sat in Biology class, tears in my eyes as the beautiful young girl stood in front of me telling her story of the car accident that almost claimed her life. I sat in awe as she talked about her recovery and her daily life, living with traumatic brain injury. Inspired by her strength and encouraged by her perseverance and determination, I had to meet this amazing girl! And she has been my best friend ever since!

I was a pre-medical student, struggling to pay for college, working full-time, and there were so many times I doubted myself, wanting to quit. Kelly would not let that happen. Kelly was there for me every step of the way, giving me encouragement, strength, and determination to never give up. Those same characteristics Kelly needed to survive and recover through her accident, she had given to me and made me who I am today. The story of Kelly's tragic accident, her struggle through recovery, and her journey to succeed provides encouragement, motivation, comfort, and strength not only for families and victims of traumatic brain injury, but for all of us who have ever had an incredible dream."

Dr. Amanda Waugh Moy, Emergency Medicine

"Kelly Bouldin Darmofal's account is unique, yet widely applicable: she teaches any who have suffered TBI—and all who love, care for, and teach them—insights that are not only novel but revolutionary.

1. *Poetry of art and science.* With her occasional poems, she opens a window into her brain, revealing that language is sometimes at its best when brief, incomplete, and thereby widely evocative of experience that is irreducible to simple sentences. Her first poem after the injury—spoken impromptu—is a gift to literati and scientists alike, who will discover what they didn't know about language and brain. Sometimes sardonic, often subtle, her rhetoric is life-giving as well as life-celebrating.

2. *Theology.* Like Job, she learned the hard lesson of a faith that ultimately made her both "thankful to my non-intervening God," as she put it, and for that reason, resolute in becoming the person she now is. Her experiences exemplify that providence can't be preached—to self or others—apart from persistent self-actualization.

3. *Education.* Warnings against inflexible educational bureaucracy abound in her descriptions of narrow-minded teaching. Yet, she recognizes good teaching so well that she becomes a teacher herself and models what all teachers must emulate: respect for students as persons in all their idiosyncratic potential. She understands mediocrity as the great millstone around the neck of education.

The book is not simply worth reading; it is necessary reading for patients, poets, professors, preachers, and teachers."

Dr. Frank Balch Wood

(Frank Wood is professor emeritus of neurology-neuropsychology at Wake Forest School of Medicine and an ordained Baptist minister.)

"Kelly was referred to me by her neurosurgeon who happened to be a close friend of mine. His and her description of her traumatic injury and the tenacity with which she fought to regain basic functional abilities was impressive at that time. Her efforts since then should be inspirational to us all. In short, one cannot measure her attributes of determination and perseverance, spirit and courage, and willingness to embrace the whole of life. The result of her efforts speaks for itself."

Dr. James D. Mattox, Jr., M.D.
Diplomate American Board of Psychiatry and Neurology

LOST IN MY MIND:

Recovering from Traumatic Brain Injury (TBI)

Kelly Bouldin Darmofal

Modern History Press

Lost In My Mind: Recovering from Traumatic Brain Injury (TBI)

Learn more at www.ImLostInMyMind.com

Published by
Modern History Press, an imprint of
Loving Healing Press
5145 Pontiac Trail
Ann Arbor, MI 48105

www.ModernHistoryPress.com
info@ModernHistoryPress.com
Tollfree USA/CAN: 888-761-6268
Fax: 734-663-6861

Distributed by Ingram Book Group (USA/CAN), Bertram's Books (UK).

First Printing: November 2014

Library of Congress Cataloging-in-Publication Data

Darmofal, Kelly Bouldin, 1977- author.
Lost in my mind : recovering from traumatic brain injury (TBI) / Kelly Bouldin Darmofal.
p. ; cm. -- (Reflections of America)
Includes bibliographical references and index.
ISBN 978-1-61599-244-7 (pbk. : alk. paper) -- ISBN 978-1-61599-245-4 (hardcover : alk. paper) -- ISBN 978-1-61599-246-1 (ebook)
I. Title. II. Series: Reflections of America series (Unnumbered)
[DNLM: 1. Brain Injuries--psychology. 2. Brain Injuries--rehabilitation. 3. Personal Narratives. WL 354]
RC451.4.B73
617.4'81044--dc23
2014020907

Cover photo by David Amundson of Superieur Photographics
Oprah Winfrey photo courtesy of Salem College.
Glamour Shots Inc. photo reproduced with permission.
First Printing: November 2014

Dedication

I dedicate this book to my dear friend Britt Armfield, who died in a car crash in June 1993 and continued to speak to me, and to Matt Gfeller, who died of TBI while playing football in August of 2008. His motto was "I won't let you down," and he didn't.

My story is also dedicated to Carolyn and Robert Bouldin—and especially to my patient husband Brad and to my son Alex, who have both provided the happy ending.

I have a dream
To race the lightning
To be the best
To race the wind
I have a dream
To race the lightning
And win!

(Kelly Bouldin, age 10)

Contents

Poems

Figures/Pictures

Foreword

This book should be required reading for people who have sustained significant head injuries and have neurological deficits and, also, especially for the families of those unfortunate individuals. This is the story of a young lady looking forward to her life with great hopes and expectations of success. She had many advantages with her family, position, and education. It is a compelling account of an individual with great determination, who gradually overcame, to a major degree, numerous struggles and frustrations that she confronted her through her recovery.

Her family's support, understanding, and encouragement played a major role in her healing and were indispensable in shepherding her through this ordeal. She received excellent professional guidance; but it was her determination and focus that played the major role in her recovery. In the end, it is an uplifting and happy conclusion to a long struggle by a very fine lady. No two individuals with head injuries are alike because of the varying degrees of injury and their pre-injury personalities. Also, their support systems are unique to them.

I would strongly recommend this book to individuals with TBI.

Dr. David L. Kelly, Jr. M.D.,
Neurosurgery Chair Emeritus
Wake Forest University

Preface

Memory is elusive even in the best of times. Kelly, who has a viable reason to have difficulty with recall, may be less guilty than I am, if errors have been made in *Lost in My Mind*. In writing journals, I was simply trying to conserve memories for my daughter—the ones I knew she might need someday. Thus writing was both therapy and conservation. In my diaries (never intended for publication), some names have been changed in the interests of privacy; sentence fragments have been completed; and tenses and/or misspellings have been altered for clarity. We both apologize if our memory of data is flawed, and if anyone deserving is omitted from this memoir.

I always told my child that putting her life back together was like a difficult jigsaw puzzle; we would focus on her healing and accept the help of others—one piece at a time. I gave my writings to Kelly after her college graduation, telling her to abridge them at need, and omit anything others would find offensive. I thank her for accepting my gift of words, and for facing her mother's personal angst. We've both given readers the truth as we knew it then and today, with no intent to belittle any organization or individual; our writings reflect the perceptions and fears we both experienced post-TBI.

Carolyn Bouldin

Prologue

A flash of pain shoots through my shoulder as I push my son's stroller toward the park nearby—the price of motherhood, I think, and one gladly paid. My son, the lucky boy, looks like his father. I look like any typical mother, shoving an overloaded stroller uphill through a neighborhood filled with oak trees and "typical" young families, like mine. Looking at me, you probably wouldn't guess I'm a survivor of TBI; that I'm disabled, often in pain, and that pushing a stroller represents a twenty-three-year victory for me—a survivor and mother, teacher, wife. I am happy today because I can push a stroller, because I can walk, and use two hands to type. The stroller, says my mother, is much like the walker I once used to relearn the skill of walking. I don't, however, remember all the details of that journey, but I'd like to share what I do remember.

Come into my home. Look carefully at the Post-it notes scattered around my den. In the kitchen, you'll notice a large chart noting, in bold black print, my son's schedule for formula feedings, for naps, for solid foods. You'll meet "the twins," two rescue mutts who love me dearly. They don't care if I can't thread a needle, or remember exactly how old they are. We are much alike, happy in the moment, forgetful of earlier ones.

Does my Pomeranian mutt Mitzy remember the day someone set her on fire? No, Mitzy and I are good at suppressing bad memories. But I remember when my husband brought her home from a kill shelter. He saved her as he saved me. Some memories do last.

Do you remember where you were in 2000 as the ball dropped in Times Square? I have no idea how I welcomed the new millennium, or the make of the car I drove that year. Can I ask, "How did it feel when you had your first real kiss?" I wish I remembered my own. But I can't even recall who my grade school teachers were, or what my prom dress looked like. Fragments of memory are all I possess of high school. Yet I will do my best to remember glimpses of my teenage years to help the reader fully embrace what it's like to have TBI as an adolescent. My story really begins in 1992 after my traumatic brain injury. That was the year I didn't die, but often wished I had. I now do research on TBI. I have lectured on the subject, and won a prestigious literary award for a TBI-inspired article in *English Journal.* Honestly, I'd rather not travel back to re-enter the torment of TBI convalescence. I don't want to tell you how similar I was to the blind man who trips on a chair someone moved from its usual position. In my house, meticulous neatness is imperative. If you move my leather coat from a hook to the closet, I may forget I own it.

As I put my son down for his nap, I wonder if someday he will mind having a slightly different mother. It's for his sake, however, that my TBI story needs to be told. Some tell me he is more likely to die from TBI than from any disease known to mankind. In 2014, posts the Centers for Disease Control and Prevention (CDC), there will be 2.5 million new victims of TBI. Not all will be soldiers and athletes—many will be children and teens. So, and I hold my breath, travel with me through a time more happily forgotten. I remember little of 1992, so my story begins with the unusual journal of my mother, Carolyn Bouldin. She wrote on greeting cards, hospital napkins, and a computer. She apologizes for any unintentional inaccuracies. This diary was written for me—if I lived and wanted memories—and not for publication.

To explain why I cannot personally write about '92, the following section is an example of my ramblings, which mother recorded three months after I was injured:

First Memories (Recorded By Carolyn Bouldin)

I'm very cold. And I'm very hungry. Mom is crying. Again. She looks funny crying, but I can't laugh. I can't cry, either. The kitchen isn't very far, so I'll make a peanut butter and jelly sandwich myself—bread from the basket, and LaLa's strawberry jelly. I spread it on the bread myself, lots and lots of jelly. And I'm very cold. My sweater should be here somewhere. Look for the sweater.

Not on the chair and not in the hall. My bedroom isn't very far. My robe is on the bed, so I put it on and look in the mirror. I look white. Mom says she is blue, but she looks pink. I can play the music myself: "I'm Alive" by Pearl Jam. Loud music now... good. Everyone says it is good to be alive, but what do they know? The phone never rings anymore. I just want to go outside by myself and take a walk and smoke a cigarette without Dad seeing me. I put on my shoes—tennis shoe on this foot, bedroom slipper on that foot. I can dial the phone and get someone to meet me. Mom is still crying. And she looks funny that way. I wish she would make me a sandwich. I'm so hungry.

My sister Tyler is talking on the phone. That's why I can't get calls from my friends. They came to the hospital because my mom said so. Tyler likes dogs but not cats. She says she does, though. She says they taste like chicken. Then she laughs. There must be a rule for what is funny, but I don't know it. People laugh all the time, and I don't know why. Maybe Tyler will cook me some chicken.

I think I was supposed to die on September 17th. But I'm going back to school instead. School will be better...

Kelly (December 1992)

Today it is hard to believe these were my actual words and thoughts. I'd think mother made this up if she didn't hate lying more than she hates large crawling spiders.

Clearly I was lost in my mind, lost within my own body, and searching for a very long time. Surviving and recovering from a traumatic brain injury can be a surreal journey involving caregivers, families, both genetic and acquired, teachers, employers, therapists, pets, and children. Fortunately, my mother saved every napkin filled with notes, every medical report, and every report card from my various schools. "Saving them helped me believe you would live," she says.

My story is at best a collage of recollections, most of which are accurate. It presents what I learned of life with TBI—a journey back from hell. I apologize for presenting early 1992 via my mother's journals, but I need her memories. I tried to begin this memoir in 2002, but my lack of memory hampered any attempt for a second page:

> As I begin to tell you what traumatic brain injury is like, please understand that I was in an automobile accident over ten years ago—September 17, 1992, to be exact. At 10:20 p.m., on a Thursday night. I cannot remember many details, so I must rely on my mother's journals and the letters and notes of doctors and friends. I do know that my fifteenth birthday came and went five days before the accident, and that I had been in high school for just three weeks. This year of '92 was destined to be an incredible year. My sister Tyler was an ACC cheerleader at Wake Forest University, and I was a cheerleader on my high school Junior Varsity squad.
>
> I was blonde, yet smart; flirtatious but not yet dating, as my parents were strict about my riding in cars with other teenagers. The football games I cheered for were on Thursday nights, which left the weekends open for following Tyler's Wake Forest squad around the country. Study time was no problem, as I learned quickly in class and made my "A's" with ease. A boy named Alex, who was a senior soccer player, was actually interested in me. And part of me hates to admit that as a high school freshman, I completely loved and admired my parents, Bob and Carolyn. Unlike most of my friends, I was rarely at war with the older generation. My mother was a high school English teacher who worked with the learning disabled. She understood teenagers better than I did at times.
>
> Now I can't remember what I wanted to say...

Part One: Excerpts from My Mother's Journal

Part One: Excerpts from My Mother's Journal (abridged) is a compilation of Carolyn Bouldin's diaries and memories of Kelly's convalescence, and is told in the mother's voice.

1 The Incident

On September 17, 1992, Kelly Vaden Bouldin left home to grab a Burger King chicken sandwich with friends. She was fifteen years old and quite hungry after cheerleading for the first JV football game of the season. Not allowed to ride with 16-year-old new drivers, our beautiful and talented Kelly left home with Zach, the 18-year-old son of family friends. She did not come home.

At 10:20 p.m., Zach turned his head to speak to Chad, a loquacious sophomore in the back seat. The road was curvy on Westview Drive near Kelly's house, and the distracted young teenager drove directly into a telephone pole. The pole, unprotected by a curb, snapped in two. Kelly was in the suicide seat of the sturdy Honda Accord. Her seatbelt was fastened, but she had pulled out of the shoulder strap to shush the rowdy backseat passenger. Five days after her fifteenth birthday, three weeks after becoming a freshman at R.J. Reynolds High School in Winston-Salem, North Carolina, Kelly suffered a traumatic brain injury—a severe closed-head injury.

I had never heard of TBI, nor did I know it was the leading cause of death for children and young adults in the U.S. (Schroeter et al., 2010). This was a fact in 1992. It is true today.

In layman's terms, Kelly hit the right frontal portion of her forehead on the dashboard of a car that severed the telephone pole. She had no other injury than a harsh blow to the head. There was no blood, yet Kelly was unconscious. The two boys were minimally affected, and they expected her to wake within moments. She did not.

Kelly was unconscious when a neighbor, Dr. Romey Fisher, pulled her from the Honda that had no air bags. She was flailing about, and had a seizure in the ambulance during the ten-minute drive to the

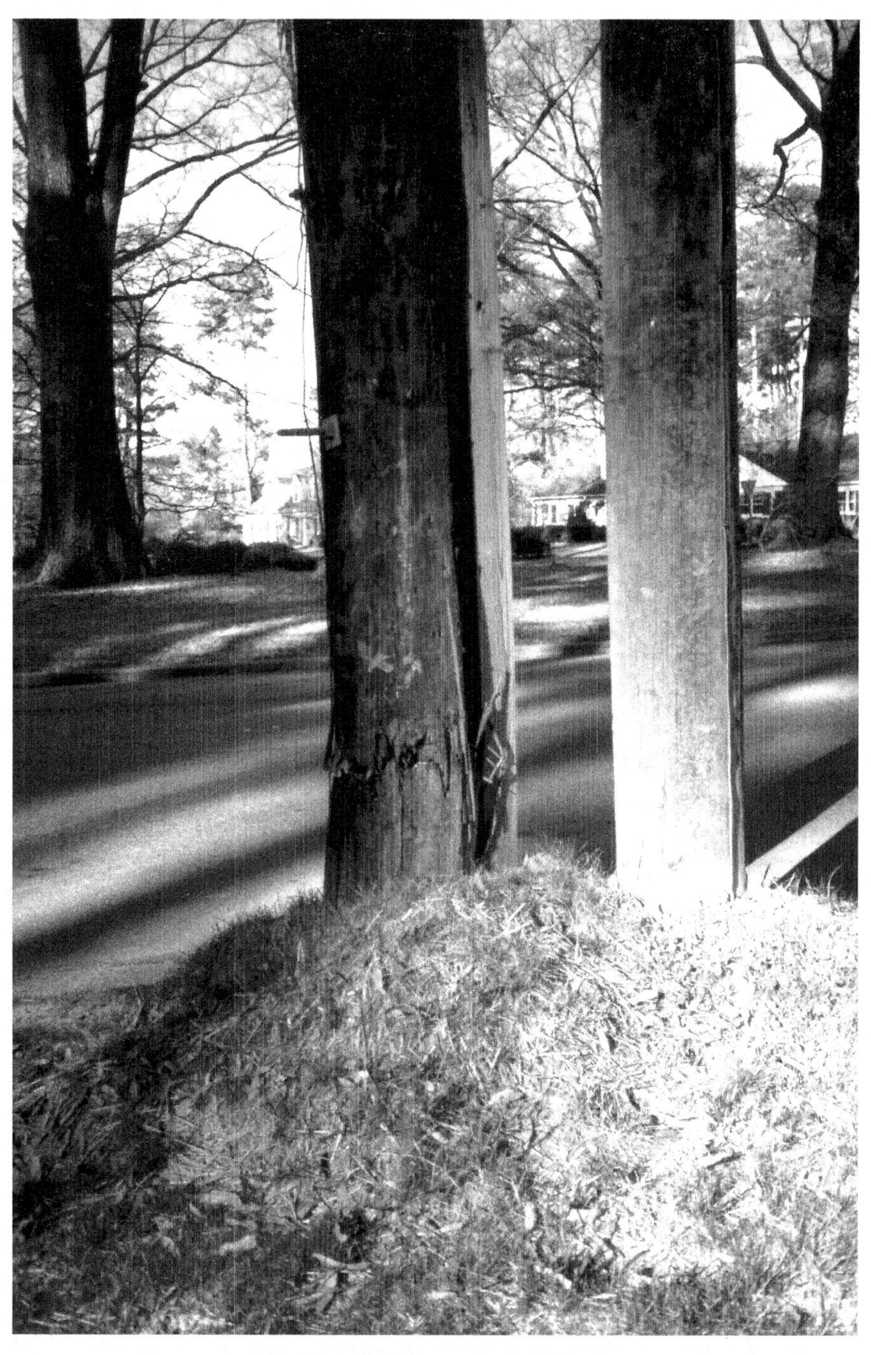

Split telephone pole (on left)

hospital. Because she was struck on the right side of her forehead, Kelly's brain had a whiplash reaction, causing injury and bleeding to the back left side of her brain. There was bleeding in the right frontal area of the impact, indeed in both frontal areas. Kelly also suffered brain stem trauma. She was hemorrhaging into every ventricle of her brain.

Thus only time would tell if my young child could awaken at all... or if she would remain in a PVS—permanent vegetative state —or die.

Kelly's injuries were quite severe, and her father and I were told she might not last the night. I still hear the echoes of the emergency room receptionists: *Does she have a living will? Is she sexually active? Why didn't she have I.D.? Has she been exposed to HIV?* "NO, NO, AND NO... she has never been on a date!" I know that any parent alive can imagine the pain and anguish that stole our daughter's childhood.

Yet, on that evening in '92, Bob and I were waiting for Kelly's return when the phone rang at about 10:22 p.m. Dr. Fisher, a close friend, advised us that our child was all right despite the fact that she and her friends had hit the telephone pole near his yard. My first statement was strangely calm, to the point: "Is she paralyzed, or blind?"

"No," Dr. Fisher answered. "The biggest problem is that she is not awake... but she probably will be when you get to the hospital."

She was not. Dr. Fisher had wisely, instantly sent Kelly's ambulance to the major trauma center at Wake Forest Baptist Medical Center. The boys, both alert, were sent to another ER at Forsyth Hospital a few miles away. Had Romey made another decision, Kelly would probably not have survived.

My husband and I arrived at the hospital at about 10:45 p.m., parked illegally and flew inside. After we had answered a myriad of insurance-related questions, we were finally given our daughter's medical status. Kelly had been placed in a medical coma, and her brain was heavily oxygenated to minimize brain swelling. A pressure monitor was inserted into her brain so that if too much swelling ensued, part of her skull would be removed to allow room for further expansion. Doctors informed us that Kelly couldn't possibly awaken for at least three days. She registered a 5 on the Glasgow Coma Scale (8 or below indicates severe brain injury).

Oh, God! My child was now in the hands of strangers—strangers devoid of smiles. I was, however, oddly calm in the surreal environment of the emergency facility. I had stepped through the looking glass that separated the "normal" world from the world of those whose lives could never again be what they expected.

Soon Dr. Fisher arrived, having tended to the more minor needs of the car's other passengers. He looked at me and wrapped me in a blanket, because I was entering a state of extreme and delayed shock. I was shaking; my teeth were chattering.

"Who should I call to come be with you?" he asked.

Winston-Salem had been my home for over 20 years. Surely I should call some friends. But who to call in the middle of the night, knowing Kelly might not live until morning. Who should be called to hold me if my child died in the night? I simply shook my head.

For some odd reason, I felt I had no right to call anyone. Such a terrible burden to share. Even my older daughter Tyler, a sophomore at Wake Forest University, shouldn't be called until morning. She could have an accident rushing to the hospital. I felt I hadn't the kind of friends I needed. I was numb. I didn't want my minister with me to tell me of God's mercies, or my parents, whose grief would make our tragedy more real. I lay beside my stunned husband on an inflated beach raft in the ICU waiting room, and existed in misery until morning, trying to imagine the woes of other mothers who had rested on that wretched plastic raft.

And I was so wrong about not calling friends. The daylight came, and Kelly was still holding on. At least sixty friends swarmed the ICU waiting area, holding me and talking to my husband, Bobby, bringing us coffee, food, strength. Kelly's story was not in the newspaper on September 18th. I had demanded of the police to withhold a press release so that Kelly's friends could learn about the news in a kinder way. But somehow they knew, and came by the scores. And they stayed. We laughed and prayed, and together we found the power to keep breathing, minute by minute.

Then another night came, and as our friends left, my strength waned, as if their leaving lessened Kelly's strength as well. I can't remember the second night.

The next day I turned to my best friend Ann Davis, and told her that I knew what would help me most. I couldn't be strong alone. Ann is a former nurse, and she mobilized the friends I didn't know I had.

Making a calendar of shifts (my treasured possession still), she kept someone with me every waking moment. Asking for this kind of help was so foreign to me, but I quickly learned that to survive the after-

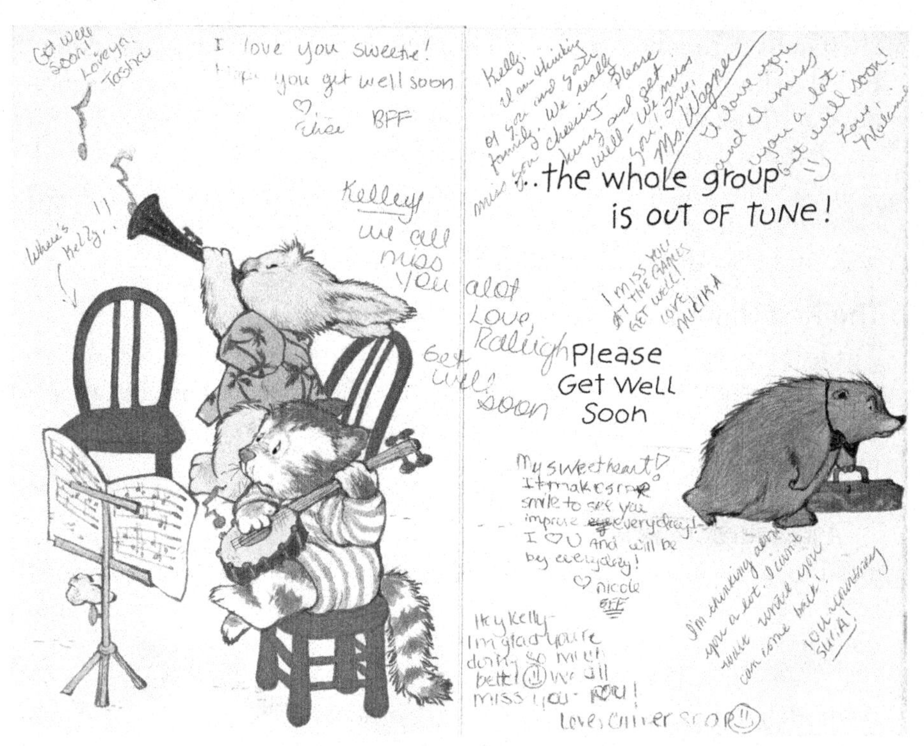

Get-Well card from friends

math of severe brain injury, my family would need a great amount of assistance. To obtain this level of support, I would have to ask for it, and others would be glad to give. I want to thank Ann, Barbara, Cynthia, LaLa, Diane, and all of the other names on that list of friends. I didn't realize that you cared so much about my child, or me.

When Dr. David Kelly told me my daughter was still alive in the dawn of September 18th, I called my daughter at Wake Forest University. I told Tyler about the wreck without crying. I did not tell her on the phone how serious Kelly's injury was. I informed her that her sister was in a coma, but that she would be okay. Kelly would probably be awake soon. I asked Tyler not to rush but to come when she could. And she did. My 19-year-old daughter was a sophomore at Wake Forest, a business major, a varsity cheerleader; yet here she was, holding me when I needed her. I met her new boyfriend. I saw him holding Tyler up while she cried uncontrollably. The boyfriend was holding Tyler up, and then she was holding me. "I'm glad he is here for her," my mind said. She asked me what she could do and I spoke:

"Go back to school and live a normal life.... Don't cancel anything. I need to know that one of us is living a normal life... I need something good to think about!"

That is what she did. Tyler kept cheering, making good grades, and visiting when she had moments to spare. I would learn later from her roommate, Julie Polson, how much Tyler cried, how devastated she was, and how difficult a time this was for her.

The Red-Haired Resident

On September 18th, my family was evidently assigned a social worker employed by Baptist Hospital. She appeared to be about twenty-two, and wore cute little suits in neutral colors. She came to see me and gave me a sideways hug.

"Mrs. Bouldin," she said, "Are you feeling depressed?"

Astounded, I made some rude rejoinder like, "No, I love hospitals and I'm just waiting to see if my child will live." Then I gave the polite response. "What do we need a social worker for?" I hemmed and coughed.

"Well, for whatever you might need," she replied. "You might need a wheelchair to take home with you or a hospital bed, and counseling is avail..."

I told her to leave at once. My mind was unable to cope with the concept of wheelchairs at this point, but she kept appearing each morning, more regularly than the doctors.

"Mrs. Bouldin, are you perhaps a little blue today?" she would ask.

I left a call for Dr. Michael McWhorter, one neurosurgeon in charge of Kelly's case, requesting that the social worker be removed from my life. And I couldn't resist asking where this girl actually went to college. She never came back.

The red-haired resident doctor wasn't as obviously objectionable. In fact, he was the first human being in the ICU to communicate with me in any depth. Surgeons are wonderful, but so busy saving lives that a resident generally appears to cover the chitchat, or at least this was our experience. This fellow told me calmly what to expect concerning Kelly's prognosis. As if he were reading from a chart, he told me that she might not live. She might need a shunt in her brain if the pressure rose and needed relieving. She might live and remain a vegetable. Lastly, she might recover up to 90% of her former capacity, eventually. I could easily see that the resident felt this was the best-case scenario.

He then warned me that I must never, ever expect to regain the Kelly I once knew. At this point, I developed antipathy for this young well-intended person, who may have been correct except for telling me what never to do.

There is an absence of hope in such a place, an utter vacuum where dim rays of light should be allowed to survive. I will never know why I was constantly discouraged from having any hope.

Meanwhile my daughter continued to sleep.

As to the resident, he reappeared daily for about a week to remind me to keep my expectations low—until I asked Dr. McWhorter to send him the way of the social worker.

Both the social worker and the resident had good intentions. However, it was not their job to lower my expectations. Every janitor, nurse, volunteer in a hospital will take an interest in a coma victim, freely giving you advice about what to do, what rehab centers are best, and so forth. After listening to every positive word I could glean from anyone, I became inexpressibly confused. One of Kelly's doctors then told me to pick one person to listen to and trust. So that is what I did. I also learned that you can trust yourself. Take the tidbits of good advice others offer, and avoid opinions that you haven't the skill to assess.

Shearing - 9/19/92

I was told early on that Kelly had suffered from brain shearing. This phenomenon cannot be measured by an MRI. In essence, the tiny neurons that connect the brain with the spinal cord are too small to be seen on X-ray. These neurons suffer a whiplash trauma during brain injury. They are stretched or broken or twisted. When a child like Kelly is young, there is good chance for the neurons to reconnect, or to form new pathways for brain signals when old ones are severed. This is a primary reason doctors cannot predict the amount or recovery for a victim of TBI—some things aren't measurable. I learned about phenomena like shearing from doctors, but mostly Kelly's nurses helped me understand her wounds and symptoms.

Doctors alerted me to a TBI filmstrip being shown twice weekly, but I was always too busy helping Kelly to attend. So I asked questions all the time. The nurses were more helpful than the neurosurgeons, who were kind but often unavailable. These remarkable women and men were encouraging, explaining that the healthier and stronger Kelly's body had been, the more likely she was to heal faster.... So all the years of soccer and dance and gymnastics could pay off after all.

Also, nurses and therapists were very alert to Kelly's pre-wreck IQ. Evidently, the higher it had been, the more likely that she would "come back." Again, I realized prior efforts like the frequent homework help from Bobby and me had not been wasted. Kelly might never make another A, but a solid student could get well faster—a probable IQ loss after a severe TBI might not prevent Kelly from having a meaningful future, some kind of a useful life.

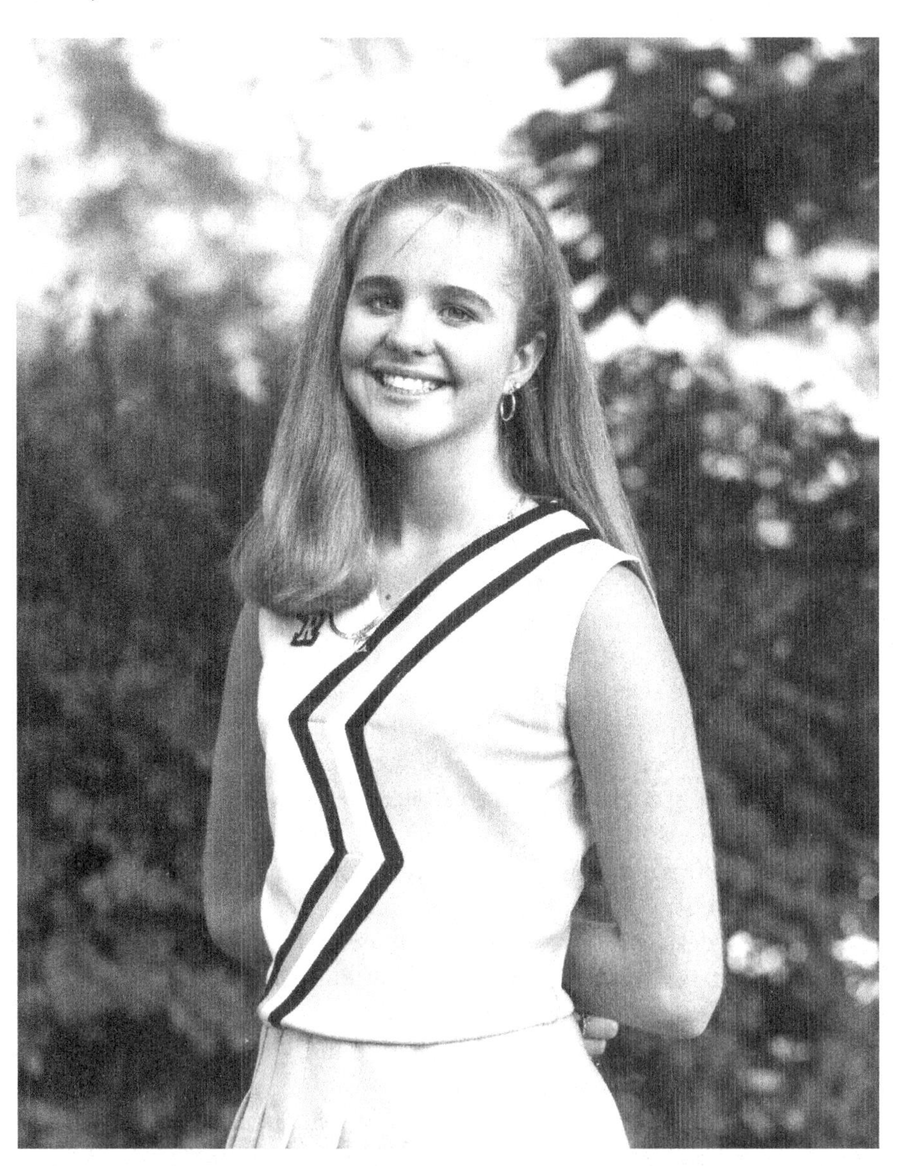

Cheerleading picture (August 1992)

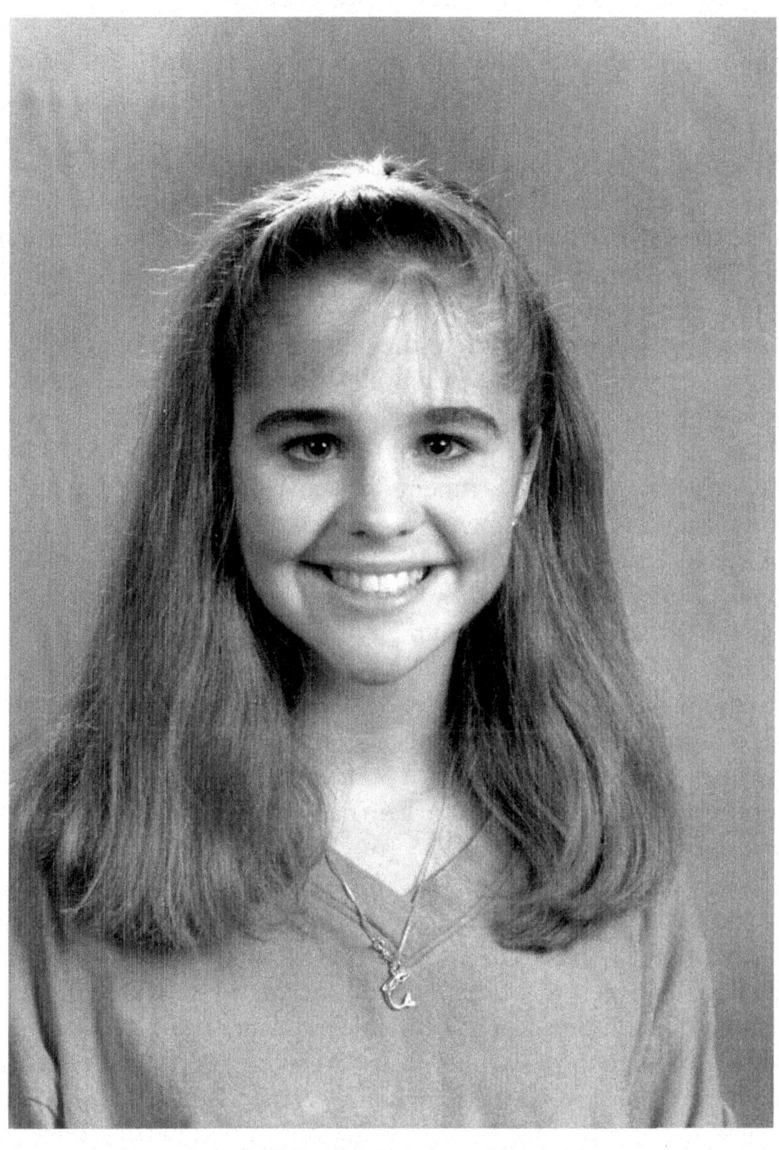

Kelly - Portrait (age 14)

Things That Helped (The First Three Days)

"Humor is the absence of terror, and terror is the absence of humor."
– Lord Buckley

The ICU nurses requested pictures of Kelly, showing her as she appeared before the car crash, to be placed above her bed. They wanted to visualize the patient they were treating as a bona fide human being, not a swollen wreck victim. With the placement of those pictures, I knew that Alice, as well as the other ICU nurses, would labor to save Kelly's life. When they combed her long blonde hair in neat French braids and requested double shifts to stay with her, I knew my daughter was in good hands. Kelly's staff of nurses kept her looking lovely, which I appreciated more than words could express. They not only spent time arranging her hair, but also shaving her legs with lotion and trimming her nails.

A black sense of humor had developed in the ICU waiting room, as Bob and I sat with at least 50 of Kelly's friends each day. Zach (who drove the car) and Chad (the loud passenger) were nursing bruises and cracked ribs, and they sat with our family and friends, waiting for Kelly to awaken. Another family, the Grays, was present in our area; they received dozens of phone calls. The phone was generally answered by whoever sat nearest, usually one of Kelly's friends, and the questions reverberated, "Anyone here named Gray? Are you Mr. Gray? Is anybody present called Gray?"

"I'm black and I'm blue... *but I'm not gray*!" Chad replied each time. I'd believed I would never laugh again, but I fell apart giggling. Later, when Kelly began to awaken, and would thrash and kick male attendants between their legs, we all became hysterical. The nurses christened her "Longlegs." Everything was so strangely funny—we allowed laughter to replace the tears everyone was afraid to release. Laughter is so good. It helps when nothing else can. I also recall laughing wildly when 14-year-old Carla discovered the doctors had to shave some of Kelly's scalp: "It will kill her," she hollered. Everyone laughed at the incongruity.

My closest friends, Barbara Price and Ann Davis, smuggled wine into a thermos and dragged me into a patio area to drink it. They actually made me laugh with their "chardonnay tea." They even ordered pizza for friends in the waiting room. These were the friends who never left me alone. Ann continued her calendar of visitors, scheduling someone to stay with me for predetermined periods of time. This one act saved my sanity. Alone, I always imagined the worst. With others, I was forced to remain an optimist. Friends who cared were essential to me.

Several friends who were nurses, therapists, and doctors helped the most. They had the medical terminology to explain what was going on with Kelly (They know you, and tell you the truth).

Comfortable and clean clothing helped. Since I wouldn't leave Kelly, I looked like a contaminated dirt lizard, and smelled like "hospital!" One friend, Ann Reagan, bought me two new warm-up suits. Wearing the new and clean clothes, I felt better, so I acted nicer to everyone.

Meeting mothers of persons with brain injuries, who had survived, helped hugely.

Going outdoors and looking at trees seemed to help my sense of permanence and stability. It felt like the trees were resting and waiting for Kelly to wake up.

Seeing the pressure monitor in Kelly's head read at "2" helped (this was a very good, low reading). Nurses let me stay with her more than visiting hours allowed. They knew she might die. Those little minutes holding her hand helped me breathe in, out, in, out.... Each one mattered.

First Purposeful Movement - 9/19/92

The monitor was removed and Kelly tried to climb out of the bed. This was Kelly's first purposeful movement, her third day in ICU. She was withdrawn from the medical coma that over-oxygenated her blood to keep the swelling in her brain down. This was both a horrible and wonderful day. When Kelly was removed from life support successfully and out of deep coma, we were warned that she might not move or breathe again on her own. Bob and I waited to see the look on the doctor's face when he left us to withdraw supports. Our friends literally held us up for those seemingly endless moments. Then we heard laughter from beyond the door. A nurse rushed into the ICU waiting room to say, "She's trying to climb off the table. That little girl wants to go home!"

Yet Kelly wasn't really awake at this time. Her eyes were closed and she did not speak, but, hallelujah, she was strong enough to kick those strangers tying her with restraints to an unfamiliar bed.

9-18-1992

Dear Kelly,

I'm not really sure where to start, but I'm sure by the time you get around to reading this, you will have figured out what's going on if you don't remember. Actually, you'll probably know alot more than I do. It was so wierd on Friday, I came to school in a good mood, and I was planning on talking with you alot. In fact, that was all I was thinking about when I saw Charlie in a clump of red-eyed, sobbing girls. When he first told me, I didn't understand it - or maybe I didn't want to. When I finally figured out, I must've been in shock or something, because for an hour after that I thought it was all some cruel joke. Mr. Alexander is going to let me take the test over we had that day, because that was only 2nd period and I was still spaced out. Everybody that knows you was either like that or crying.

God, I don't mean to depress you, its just that I like you alot - we all do. I wanted to stop by and see you this weekend, I really did, but I was in the mountains with my dad all weekend. I hope you're up soon enough to see the carnation I bought you at school for homecoming, before it wilts or something. Anyway, your room probably looks like a jungle by now from all of the flowers and stuff. I know I haven't known you for long, and you probably think I'm wierd to be this workedup about it, but I do really miss you.

Letter from a friend (09/18/92)

Day Four - 9/20/92

Kelly developed a staph infection at the IV insertion point on her right wrist. A lot of swelling… Kelly's temperature rose to 105 degrees. She was now twice critical. I do not want to write about this irony, that we might lose her not to a TBI, but to infection. The ICU nurses didn't immediately note the infection. Another visitor, Elizabeth (and another former nurse) lifted Kelly's sheet and examined her IV lines. Elizabeth saw the red, swollen right arm, which had grown to the size of a football, and alerted the hospital staff.

Day Ten - 9/26/92

Too busy to write the past few days. Today Kelly was better and her eyes, her amazing eyes, were flickering open... shut... open... fever going down...

The Boy in ICU - 9/27/92

On Kelly's 11th day in the Baptist ICU, she appeared to be napping. Earlier she'd been looking at me, and I had told and retold her about her accident, but it didn't seem to register. My friend Margaret Mills, a former nurse, admonished me to talk to her constantly, because "people in a coma can hear you, even if they can't remember what you've said."

Taking Margaret's advice, I talked and talked until no more words would come out. I played pop music, mostly Pearl Jam, for Kelly via earphones, hoping she could hear. Now Kelly was resting, and the boy in the bed next to her was, too.

Suddenly he began to seize. He writhed and twisted, and several attendants rushed to his side. The boy was dying, and I was sitting there, watching without too much emotion. I felt I existed numbly in an unfamiliar world where tragedy was commonplace.

And then I looked at Kelly. She was awake and her eyes were transfixed, wide with horror, staring at this boy as he fought for a few dying breaths. I screamed for a nurse and said, "Please believe me, she can see what's going on, and understand it!" The nurse took one look at Kelly's eyes and drew curtains around us, blocking the view of impending death. Soon Dr. McWhorter came to check on Kelly and I told him, "She knows!"

"Then it's time to take her out of the ICU," he responded, sending Kelly on the next leg of her journey.

Kelly was moved out of ICU on September 28, and I was so happy to leave—for about ten minutes. Then I realized how completely I had relied on the 24-hour care in the ICU. Kelly's new room was directly across from the nurses' station; yet I was terrified to be totally in charge of her. She was still technically in coma even though her eyes were now open—awake but not always aware. Long periods of time passed before anyone came to check on her. I then realized, for the first time, that I would be her primary lifeline for the months and years to come.

Day Twelve and Lingerie - 9/28/92

Today was Kelly's first day out of the ICU, and I was exhausted. She still hadn't spoken, but sometimes smiled at me; she knew who I was and hugged back when I released her arms from the restraints.

I was tired in my soul. A nurse came by and handed me a bag that contained Kelly's possessions taken from her the first night in the ER.

"Go home and sleep," the nurse begged. So I left Kelly with my sister-in-law and cautiously began the drive home for a shower.

I hit a dog. It was a black lab puppy. Somewhere out of the darkness a beautiful puppy dashed out in front of my car. I stopped and found the owner. The dog was barely hurt, but I wasn't sure I should drive a car anymore.

I took a long shower, huddled up in my warmest robe, and flopped on Kelly's bed. For a brief moment, I pretended she was well and coming home any minute to blast her stereo. Then I looked up and saw the bag from the hospital. Like a Christmas present, the parcel contained reminders of my child when she was unscarred and healthy. Excited, I dumped the bag's contents onto Kelly's bed.

A lifetime ago (two weeks), I gave Kelly her first set of "fancy" lingerie for her 15th birthday. A black lacy bra was her favorite gift, and now it came back to haunt me. What I now saw on the bedspread was a bunch of tattered remnants—shreds of the clothing cut off of my child in the emergency room. Her favorite "slickies" (black gym shorts) were in pieces; the undergarments of slivered black lace that had once clung to her body were unrecognizable. Everything was cut into pieces, like my life, like hers.

The tears I had not yet shed came to me now. The pieces of lace had lost Kelly's smell. I knew I would never cry this hard again.

Why did the hospital give these fragments back to me? Why did I allow Kelly to go out that night barefoot and with no ID? I am in hell. So is she.

Saturday at Brenner Children's Hospital (WF/BMC) - 10/3/92

Today made me want to stop breathing. My sister Clara, nicknamed LaLa, came every weekend to keep me sane, more or less. She held back my despair, because caretakers need their own caretakers. The first Saturday out of ICU, we put Kelly in a wheelchair and rolled her into the recreation room of Brenner's. We turned on MTV and blasted rock and roll music. Kelly stared at the television but didn't really register what was playing. She just stared into space. She didn't react to the music, but drooled from the left side of her face, the frozen side. It was grim. LaLa and I held each other up. People don't visit much on Saturdays. Doctors don't come much. There was no therapy on the weekends, and minutes could seem like hours. So much time wasted.

When she can speak, maybe doctors will come and say she is "out of coma."

2 First Word

It was October of 1992 and my child had been in a coma for over two weeks, and on that day, she did the most commonplace thing in a teenager's life. She answered the telephone that was attached to her hospital bed. She said... "HEY!" With a feeding tube still down her throat, Kelly spoke her first word. I do not know who was more excited—me, or Dr. McWhorter, who has been quite concerned that Kelly had opened her eyes days ago, but couldn't speak one tiny syllable. Hope! I knew she would talk. My irrepressible motor-mouthed child was not going to remain in a world of silence. I told them she would speak, and she told me with her eyes. She was coming back to us as fast as she could. Dear Lord, it is hard to be patient!

The next day, Kelly's friend Mark Giordano brought us a poem he had written, in which he tried to see through her confused eyes:

> Encountered by the mural that haunts her
> Disclosed to the accounts of man
> Spirited by her love untouched
> Exposed to a stupor hidden mutually.
> Worthy of details yet not enchanted
> The altar is replenished, modifying concern
> Allowing her to descend into the age
> For she is awake, she is awake.

Mark didn't realize that it wasn't the beauty of his poem that spoke to me. It was his optimism. He believed. He told me the poem "sums up what is going on in her mind and in ours. Her mural is going away." If Mark can believe in her future, so can I.

More Firsts

I couldn't write much at the time Kelly first moved on day three, and first opened her eyes days later. The eleven days she spent in ICU left me paralyzed with fear.

It seemed longer than a week since Kelly's eyelids fluttered and I saw her blue eyes staring at me. A tiny sweet grin spread across her betubed face, the most precious smile in the world. I saw recognition in her eyes and threw my arms around her. She struggled with her arms, and the nurse released her right arm from the restraint. She hugged my neck tightly, and then patted me gently on the back. It was as if she was comforting me and saying, "I'm fine. Don't worry about me!" Naturally the doctors wouldn't agree that she recognized her mother, as patting is reflexive. But a parent knows. Bobby was there, too. Daddy got his hug as well, and perhaps breathed for the first time in a millennium.

Tears of a Father

My husband had not yet cried. He was stoic until he found Britt's letter lodged in our back door. Britt Armfield, a sophomore friend, had not yet been to the hospital, but left us this letter:

> Dear Mr. and Mrs. Bouldin,
>
> I write this letter with a certain amount of regret. I regret the fact I do not have the strength to go to see Kelly. Personally, I have gone through two open heart surgeries and a number of minor procedures, and due to that, hospitals frighten me. However, I want you to know, and Kelly to know that I love her very much and I want to see her. I pray for her every night. I pray for you both and for Tyler. I cannot imagine being thrown into the position you are in. I know Kelly is going to be okay. I know you hear that all the time; but from the bottom of my heart, for what it is worth, I want you to hear it from me. I can remember the first time I met Kelly. It was around Christmas two years ago. She had just gotten a makeover. I knew then she was a beautiful girl on the outside and through the past two years, I have come to realize she is just as beautiful on the inside.
>
> We cannot begin to answer why this happened. But God has a strange ways of doing things and there is a reason. You may never realize the reason for this, but there is one. I want you to know that I feel for you deeply. I also want you to know that I

am praying for you and I can only begin to tell you how much I hope all of our prayers will be answered. I truly wish God will comfort you and lay his healing hand upon Kelly because that is how I see her now, resting in God's hands, his eyes watching over her day and night, healing her constantly.

In Him, Britt Armfield

PS – After Kelly recovers, please let her know I was thinking of her. It would mean a lot.

"I consider that our present sufferings are not worth comparing with the glory that will be revealed in us."

– Romans 8:18, *NIV*

My husband handed me this letter in Kelly's hospital room and said, "I finally cried. And it took the words of a teenage boy I don't even know."

Karen Fry

Karen Fry was a 27-year-old mother of two, who resided next door to Kelly on the 7th floor of Brenner's. I am not sure why she had been placed in the children's section of the hospital, but Karen was in a coma much like Kelly's. She also had other injuries that made her prognosis for recovery extremely dim. I don't know if her head injury was open or closed, but I do recall her devoted young husband.

Mr. Fry spoke to me every day from September 28th until October 22nd, when Kelly left Brenner's Hospital for Myers Lake Rehab. He asked my permission to come in and watch Kelly in her various stages of recovery. Mr. Fry wanted to watch as she began to speak, walk with assistance, make a phone call, and attain other firsts. I often looked in on Karen and her poor young husband, as he stared at his comatose wife. He told me how much his children missed their mother. He did not expect her to awaken, but "in case she does, I want to watch Kelly to know what to expect next," he said. He, like me, did not know what came next. Paul Fry often walked with me as I rolled Kelly's wheelchair to therapy sessions.

"I wish I could believe Karen would ever sit up in a wheelchair," he lamented. He gave me a reality check. I had been so upset to view my own child in a wheelchair that I hadn't considered the alternative.

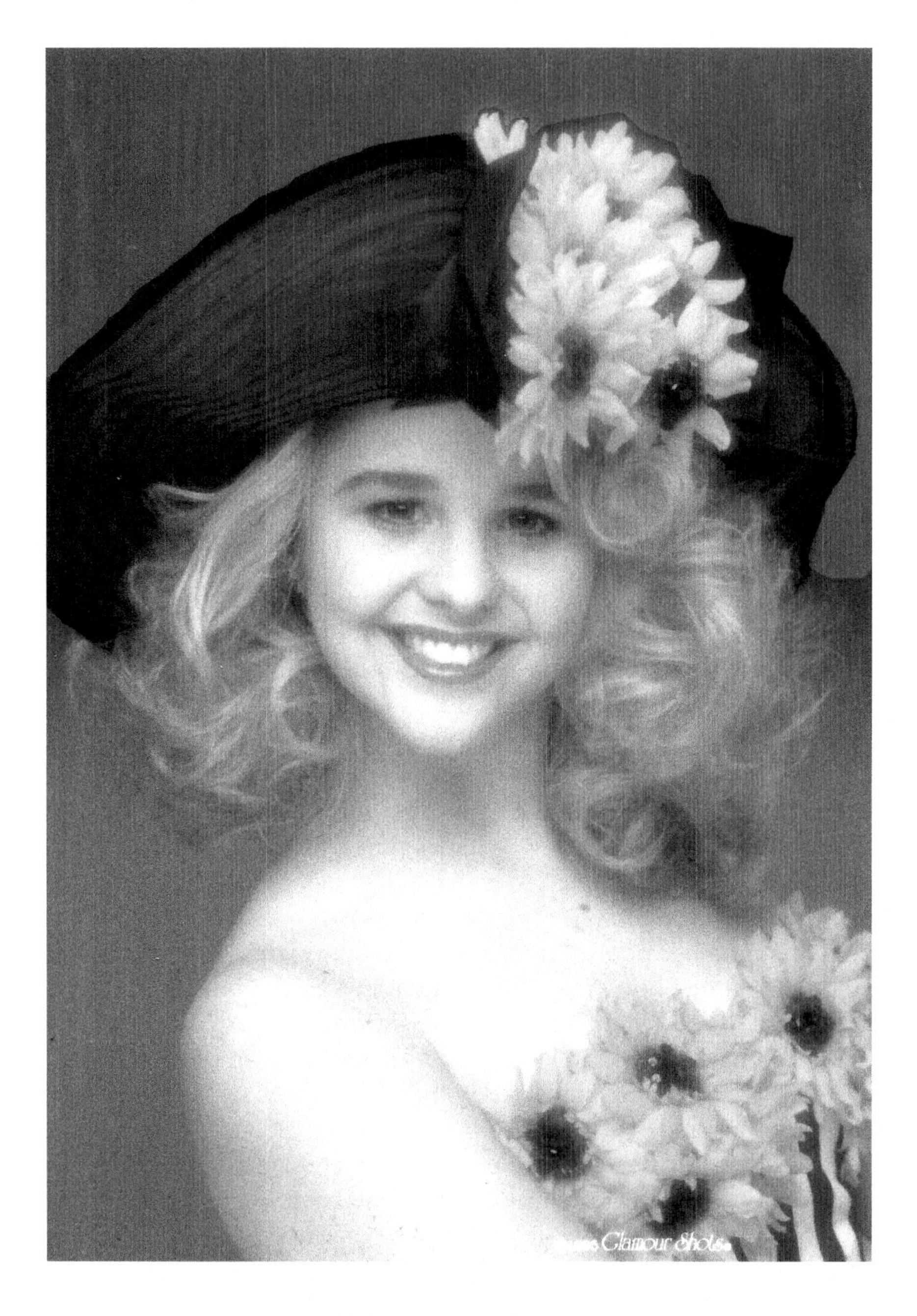

Kelly after a makeover

(One year later as I was walking through Hanes Mall, an elderly couple approached me. "Are you Kelly's mother?" the lady asked. When I said yes, she hugged me and said, "Karen Fry got her driver's license today. I'm her mother, and I thought you'd want to know." Hope. There it was again.)

Heather and a Miracle

Kelly had a room directly across from the nurse's station on the 7th floor of the hospital. Heather, a Canadian nurse, kept the more watchful eye on my child, but she didn't like me. And who could blame her? I yelled at her constantly, and nothing she did was ever fast enough or good enough. I refused to let her bathe my child. One day I climbed into the large bathing tub with my clothes still on, holding Kelly beneath her armpits. I was afraid Heather would bump her head on the faucet as another nurse had done.

And Heather couldn't stand me for another reason. I had become totally selfish. Christy Barrett was another teenager admitted to Brenner's with a TBI and multiple broken bones. Christy's head injury was open, not closed, and she had just come from surgery. Heather wanted me to give Kelly's room to Christy, who was having multiple seizures. I could see Christy seizing and the nurses running. They didn't think that Christy would live another day. The nurses wanted her room to be across from the nurses' station so that they could come to her aid immediately. I said, "No, this is Kelly's room!"

I must have subconsciously felt that if Kelly was moved to a more remote room, the nurses might forget about her. This thought was of course irrational, but it felt all too real. Playing on my guilt, the nursing staff eventually won. As we began our evacuation, I watched Mrs. Barrett faint and fall to the floor. I laughed, thinking that I never fainted so I must be stronger. I may have allowed the room trade, but I was furious. What was I becoming? I didn't feel anything for the Barretts but anger. They stole Kelly's room!

Later that day Kelly was taken to her therapy sessions in a wheel chair and, for the first time, a magic marker and paper pad were placed in her hands. She grabbed them and wrote a whole and complete sentence, "I'M LOST IN MY MIND."

Kelly is alive in there, I thought. Kelly is coming back to us, and she knows something horribly wrong is going on, but she is fighting. Kelly is here!

The day before Kelly's written sentence, I met a woman whose teenager came to therapy here. Her daughter was the victim of a burst brain aneurism in 1991. The teenager told me to keep right on hoping. I asked what she had learned that day.

"To write a complete sentence," she replied. *Wow*, I thought, *my child had already done that very thing.*

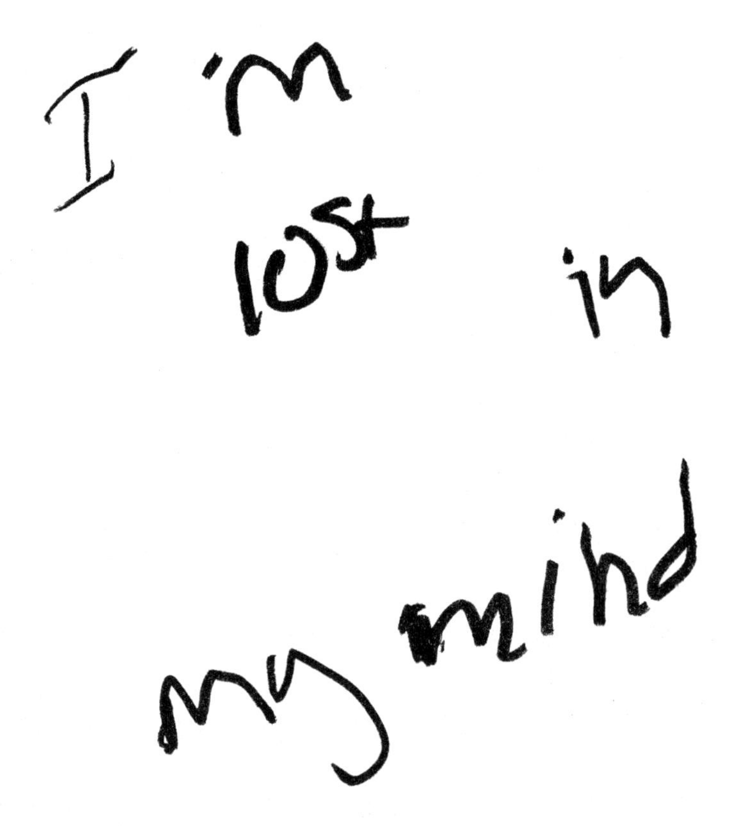

Kelly's first written sentence

Double-Jointed, Double Vision

For two weeks, I'd prayed for my daughter to move with purposeful motion. Today, week three, I take that back. Kelly is double-jointed, and her toes were causing us trouble! After a severe closed-head injury, any muscles in the body can be in paralysis. Kelly couldn't swallow safely and had a feeding tube that went down her throat into her stomach. Her arms were in restraints to keep her from jerking out the uncomfortable tube that nourished her.

Today I nodded off, and she bent her feet upwards and her toes grasped the offending tube, jerking it out and sending it onto the floor. The noise woke me from my reverie, and I immediately called her nurse. I was then forced to endure the awful sight of a team reinsert the tube as Kelly flailed.

Someday I may find this funny. My mother Evelyn said that all things can be laughed at eventually; however, I don't think this is what she had in mind. This was about as much fun as watching the medical staff jab needles into Kelly's bruised veins. I did laugh when she kicked a male nurse in the crotch. He came in to help replace her feeding tube. Even though Kelly's arms were in restraints, I would not allow them to restrain her legs, too. She constantly fought to free her arms, and I couldn't blame her. She didn't know or understand what was happening to her body, but she was in there, and she was trying so hard!

First Spoken Sentence

I'd been told that speech was part of the medical method of determining coma. Evidently, the Glasgow Coma Scale measures three things: verbal response, motor response, and visual response. Kelly's nurse told me Dr. McWhorter, trying to assess the verbal part of this scale, asked Kelly to count from one to ten. Kelly mumbled, "uno, dos, tres, quatro, cinco, seis, siete, ocho, nueve...diez." The doctor said, "She's not making sense. I'm worried."

"She sure is," said the nurse. "She's counting in Spanish!" Shortly thereafter, her first spoken sentence was "DON'T TIE ME UP!" regarding her leg restraints. Therapists were working with Kelly's writing, speech, and movement every weekday. Some felt her convalescence was time-limited... the implications of this were terrifying.

Perseverance/Perseverating

Kelly's speech therapist, Lillian, presented me with evidence of per*sev*erance or per*sev*eration. I'd been told Kelly would repeat things, or "persevere", like a broken record. Yet I saw the true impact of such behavior when Kelly began to write with paper and pencil. When asked to write the numbers one to ten, she would repeat a number. The same thing applied to the days of the week: "Monday, Tuesday, Wednesday... Monday, Tuesday..." Kelly "snagged" mentally on one word or idea and repeated it when speaking or writing.

List 10 words that begin with the letter T. T!

trip
travel
traveled
trolly
trippled
triple
try.
train
tripled
try

Words that start with T, perseverance (Kelly writing)

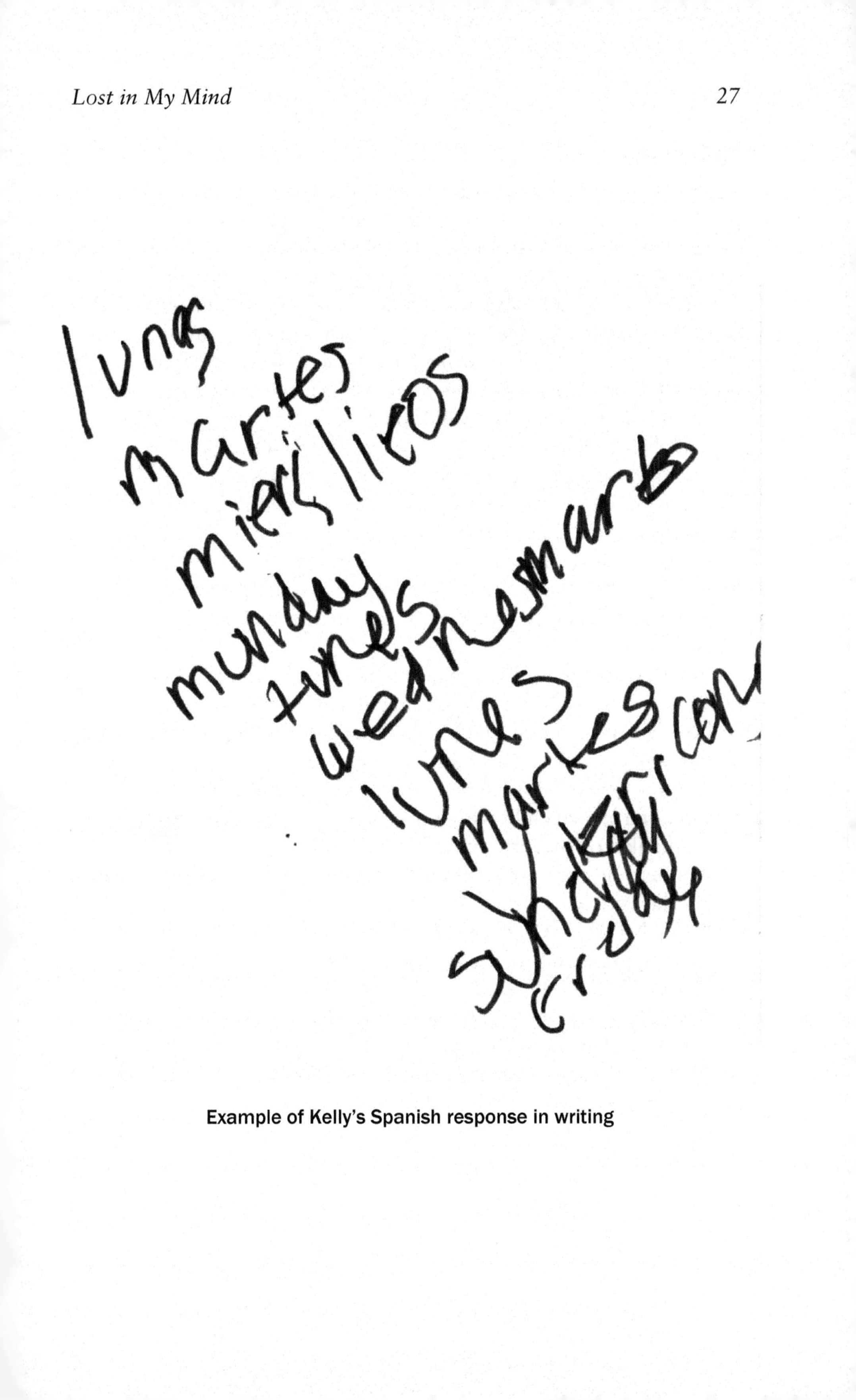

Example of Kelly's Spanish response in writing

Pam Pyrtle

Out of mistakes comes discovery. I fell asleep again and let Kelly pull out her feeding tube and her IV. Bobby hired a young woman named Pam to stay with Kelly from midnight until 7 a.m. She would stay awake so that I could go home, take a shower, and rest for a few uninterrupted hours. My sister-in-law Cynthia Bouldin would stay from 11 p.m. until Pam came, simply to extend my breathing time.

Today we received the excellent news that Kelly started her monthly period. The doctors agreed this was the biggest positive sign yet. Now we knew that Kelly's body could function normally in the future. We had all needed positive news and this certainly sufficed.

That night was going to be my first away from Kelly, and I shook at the wheel of the car going home (but I managed to avoid all dogs). Once inside, my answering machine was filled with messages. I listened, erased them, and put an outgoing message on the machine. "Kelly is better today. Her eyes are open and she is listening to television. Check in tomorrow night for an update. Sorry I can't return all messages."

The next morning, Pam gave me the one gift I didn't know I had needed! Kelly was no longer wearing diapers. Pam left me a note:

"Got Kelly up and placed her on the toilet. She went on cue. I think she remembers what to do now."

I didn't realize until that moment what a huge fear I had. The thought of a grown child who wore diapers frightened me to the core. Now, thanks to Pam, this wouldn't happen.

Pam left another note: "I went to the bathroom and Kelly called 911." She said:

"I WANT TO GO HOME."

"Where are you?" asked the dispatcher.

"I DON'T KNOW. BUT I WANT TO GO HOME!"

The nurses were still laughing about Kelly's call when I arrived at 7 a.m. They had grabbed the phone away, but were so happy she could make that call! Our family is grateful to Pam Pyrtle for keeping us constantly posted on Kelly's nightly activities.

10-9-92 11p-7a

Kelly slept all nite.
I kept the blanket on
her & the heat about
78°. She wouldn't
keep her socks on, she
kept pulling one off.
She didn't touch her
NG tube at all. I hope
you have a nice weekend
& see you tomorrow.

10-10-92

Kelly has been real restless
tonite. The nurses had to
restrain her, she kept pulling
at her tube. When she quieted
down I took the restraints
off. She got so restless
she tried to bite me.

Note from night nurse Pam Pyrtle

The Diamond

When Kelly was admitted to the ER, she was wearing an early birthday gift. I had given her a ½ carat diamond to wear in her double pierced, left ear. I had split my wedding earrings, giving each daughter one stone. Shortly after Kelly began to speak, but before she could verbalize many syllables, my husband asked me what had become of the diamond. I told him that it was not in Kelly's ear when I first saw her. "It probably fell out during the wreck, or someone cleaning her up decided to keep it," I answered. Suddenly we heard a low-pitched voice.

"Kill them!" Kelly growled in a low soft tone. We laughed and rejoiced. She was following our conversation while we thought she was sleeping. Her logic confirmed our prayer that she understood our words and explanations.

Invading the OR, Thumb Wrestling

Today I walked into an operating room and got in trouble. Kelly pulled out her IV again with her toes, and a nurse jabbed her bruised arm three times trying to reinsert it. *This shouldn't be happening*, I thought. I needed to talk to Dr. McWhorter. I walked straight into the Operating Room to find him, because it now seemed he only rarely checked in on Kelly. The entire nursing staff screamed at me, but McWhorter came to the room two hours later. He promised to have a doctor insert her IVs in the future, and again voiced his concern about Kelly's slow progress (I wish he would say something positive on occasion).

Later Zach, Mike, and Chad all came by to visit. Those were the three boys occupying the free time of the nursing staff with a betting pool. The nurses were betting on who gets to be Kelly's boyfriend. Mike Sellars was a 16-year-old who had a major crush on Kelly. Anyway, Zach and Kelly used to thumb wrestle, and today Zach held out this thumb. Kelly responded, wiggled her thumb, and he let her win. She blessed him with a huge smile. His mental state was recovering slowly like Kelly, and about at her speed.

Earlier today a friend, mother of Michael Rogers, gave Kelly a flip-and-erase pad. She told her to write the name of her boyfriend. Kelly looked up at me confused, because she didn't really have one. I had a decision to make. If I asked her to write Chad, I would make a worried boy pretty happy. Zach was simply a friend; however, if I asked her to write Mike, she might pay attention to her actions and perk up a little.

Mike Sellars was one of those boys who called Kelly often (she wasn't allowed to date yet), but she was scared of his affection. At this point, I thought, a little healthy fear might be in order.

"Write Mike," I said to her, and she did. She wrote a perfect M – I – K – E! Her eyes looked really alert for the first time all day, and I had learned something about high motivation and fear for arousing my child from a semi-permanent slumber. Mike told her "I am your boyfriend." Kelly's eyes looking up at him resembled large blue plates.

Nurses of those with brain injuries use a phrase, "The light is on!" or, conversely, "The light's not on." They are referring to the focused gaze of a patient's eyes, and some victims of TBI never really turn on their light ever again. Kelly's lights were often on when she was excited or afraid, and off when relaxed. I thought to myself that I needed to bring Christian Slater (or a similar movie star that Kelly would probably remember) to her hospital room to stimulate her light.

Halloween Coming

Our friend Nancy Lynn came to see Kelly yesterday and strung jack-o-lantern lights around the room for something fun to look at. As I stared at those lights, I began to pray for the first time since before my world was turned upside-down. My mother had always said to me, "Carolyn, prayer isn't supposed to be focused outward to the sky. Look inward, and have a deep conversation with yourself. Whatever part of God that is in you, you were born with. Find that, and it will help you to connect to the best part of others."

Daughter, I am connected, and I am asking for one wish. I'm wishing for you to recover, and live a complete life. This will be my last wish, and I will draw upon whatever forces I have in me to help all of your dreams come true.

I have not yet been able to feel the presence of God in this place. I refuse to accept any god who splatters children across highways. How can such obscenity be part of any divine plan? The only alternative is a God who believes in free will. That you, Kelly, chose to ride in that car of your own free will, and that you will fight your way back using the same free will. And God will be with you the entire way.

Dr. David Kelly once told us that "If you can endure two years of Hell, this can all be a memory!" That was an exaggeration, but the statement echoed in my brain every day. A memory? Just the hope of things possibly improving helped Kelly and me get out of bed each morning.

Fright

At Brenner's, Kelly sometimes had therapy in her room. One speech therapist, June, crawled on top of her, physically made her focus, and pushed her mouth into position around the NG tube. This wonderful girl helped Kelly breathe the words "I... love... you." Then one day, June pulled me into a corridor and said, "I could lose my job for this, but Dr. McWhorter is wrong to keep Kelly in this hospital so long. She needs 24-hour rehab now. Today!"

I said, "Why?"

She replied, "Well, if you don't hurry and go, you'll wake up one night a year from now. Kelly will be standing in a closet trying to escape the house, and she'll be screaming! So don't wait any longer. She needs more intensive help. Time is running out for her."

I was being asked to practice medicine, every single day. Did Kelly need pain meds? She couldn't tell me... and what quality of rehab?? I had to trust Dr. McWhorter.

Captain America

Mark Giordano was one of several seniors to spend a great deal of time visiting Kelly, and Mark managed to keep us laughing through the MRIs and IVs, and other grim acronyms. He and a friend, Cooper Williams, dressed up in tights and capes, yelling "It's Captain America!" as they ran through the hallways of the hospital. Kelly heard them coming.

"It's Mark!" She managed to slur around her feeding tube as he burst into her room. An American flag on his bag, "Captain America" swept into the doorway and hugged Kelly. He then did a little dance, and zoomed out again as fast as he had appeared. Later that night, Mark returned clad in his usual jeans and backwards-facing baseball cap.

"What name is on my cap, Kelly?" he asked.

"Braves," she managed to reply.

"Okay, I'm coming back in the morning. When I get here, you better be able to remember the name on my cap!" Then Mark vanished into the halls once again.

The next morning, at 6:10, Mark popped his head into Kelly's room. He woke her up. "What was the name on my cap, Kelly?"

"Braves," she answered. This was the first time Kelly had remembered a concrete fact from one day to the next. Hope, hope, and kudos to her memorable Captain!

The Birthday Present

Kelly was beginning to talk more, and she said whatever came to her mind. She thought it was her birthday, which actually was five days prior to the accident.

"Where are my presents?" she asked Mike.

"What do you want?" he questioned.

"Something EXPENSIVE!" Kelly candidly declared.

The next day, Mike placed a heavy silver chain around her neck. It looked huge on Kelly, whose 5'4" frame had shrunk to 99 pounds. We laughed a lot, and laughed more when the nurse handed Kelly her black hairbrush. The staff wanted Kelly to learn to care for herself again. Kelly pointed the brush at the TV above her bed, and tried to "click" it. It did resemble a remote control, but I began to wonder about her vision.

I held up a ball and said, "Catch this with *two* hands!" Kelly held up a single hand and I pondered a minute. "Can you hold up *four* hands?" I joked. Kelly held up two, almost pulling out her IV. Her two hands appeared to her as four...one appeared as two. Double vision, they say, is common with TBI victims

(Later we would discover that Kelly could hide her poor eyesight. Had the depth of her problem been noted sooner, she would have been spared years of torture. Many problems we blamed on "low IQ" were actually caused by lack of vision. "But I didn't remember what normal vision was like!" Kelly explained after surgery on both eyes much later).

3 Choosing a Rehabilitation Center

Dr. Michael McWhorter had intimated to me that Kelly would need to go to a rehabilitation center following her month in the hospital. Looking back, I am quite sure that he "suggested" rather than ordered this, knowing how difficult it would be for our whole family to leave our support network behind; we were allowed to accept this necessity gradually.

Finally, about the twentieth day of Kelly's ordeal, my sister Clara came to stay with Kelly while Bob and I drove to look at rehab centers. Leaving her for an entire day was one of the hardest things I have ever done. Clara promised me that if I died on the highway, she would quit her job as a college librarian and care exclusively for Kelly. I cannot express how fearful I was of becoming unable to care for my child, who so desperately needed constant care. First we traveled to Durham, NC, to see a highly recommended facility that was pristine, clean, quiet. I was told that I wouldn't be allowed to accompany Kelly for the weeks of her stay. As I walked ghost-like through the facility, it became obvious that few patients we saw there were cognizant of their environment. Kelly, on the other hand, was now sufficiently awake to be aware, and to experience fear of the unfamiliar. My decision was simple and swift. Kelly, age fifteen, would go nowhere without her mother. I am still shocked that any possible interference I might have presented to her therapists could have seemed more important than her state of mind, which would have been horrible were she torn from the comfort of her loved ones all at once.

Secondly, Bob and I visited Greensboro, NC, to view another facility. Same story. Many patients barely living. No family included. We moved on.

When we reached Myers Lake Rehab[1] in Charlotte, NC, we thought we'd stepped into Disney World. Instead of cool linoleum, we stepped onto orange wall-to-wall carpets. Instead of hospital silence, we heard laughter, conversations, sometimes irritated hollering. We saw families together, and huge therapy rooms filled with people of all ages working on various skills. We saw a high-stimulus environment, with a swimming pool and recreation facilities. And I was not only permitted to come, I was encouraged to stay with my daughter and become an active part of her recovery. Dr. McDonald seemed nice enough, and the therapists were young, energetic, and attractive. We concluded that if outpatient therapy was ruled out for her, we would travel to Charlotte.

Really Going to Rehab

I returned from visiting Myers Lake Rehab not really believing Kelly would ever need to leave home for therapy. She smiled at me when I entered her room, and I released her wrist restraints. She hugged me, pulling me closer to her. I could never take her away from the numerous friends who came to tell her school stories every day after school, even when she wasn't listening.

Days later, a woman from Myers Lake Rehab came to Kelly's room to tell us they were prepared to transport her there the next day. Dr. McWhorter, who'd promised me I wouldn't have to make a decision alone (concerning in- or outpatient therapy), was in Florida at a conference. I was furious! How could I know what to do?

I tracked down our doctor at a Florida resort. Abashed, he told me that if Kelly were his own child, he would send her to in-patient rehab. My blood turned to ice water. I signed the appropriate forms. Then I had to tell Kelly, who was, at day 34, fairly aware from moment to moment, we were going to leave home. We were leaving all of our friends, relatives, attention. She said *"No!"*

We left on October 22, thirty-five days after her accident. Lifting Kelly into the back seat of our car, sheltering her now light-sensitive eyes with sunglasses, we drove away to enter the locked ward for patients with TBI at Myers Lake Rehab. Discarding the idea of a quick visit to our home, which would have tortured us all, we took her where we hoped she would learn to walk again unassisted. At this time, Kelly was still wheelchair-reliant.

---

[1] The name of this facility has been changed for purposes of this narrative.

Things that Scared Me Most

I wish to thank the wonderful hospital staff who undeniably saved Kelly's life, but numerous things frightened me during the first month of her hospitalization. First, no one told me immediately where she was. I finally found Kelly on life support. Then the staff dodging or refusing to answer my questions frightened my husband and me. When I finally received brief answers, they contained so little hope.

I remember asking many people for an accurate explanation of TBI or the prognosis of severe closed-head injury. No one answered this question clearly either, because there was no way to ascertain what the future might hold for my daughter. I think I was most frightened by:

- People who asked to bring a priest to give my daughter last rites (Kelly is Protestant)
- Doctors who cried while visiting my child
- Social workers and staff who implied the certainty of permanent disability
- Watching the brain pressure monitor as it rose then lowered and rose again
- Neglect (perceived) from busy nurses who failed to quickly discover the staph infection my daughter had in the ICU... seeing her temperature rise to 105 degrees
- Watching other ICU victims die from seizures and gunshot wounds
- The transition from ICU to private room care, having less direct access to the nursing staff
- Insufficient contact with my child's primary doctors
- Deciding between inpatient and outpatient rehabilitation, and having to choose the best facility with little guidance from doctors or hospital staff
- Conflicting advice from doctors and therapists. Often I was asked which medication or treatment I preferred; I was asked to practice medicine on my own child on a daily basis.
- Posturing. This is when a victim' arms and legs flail about or contract in purposeless motion.
- Distinguishing between purposeless and purposeful movement and not having anyone believe I had the knowledge to

recognize the difference. For example, when my comatose child made a Vulcan salute in response to my nephew Marc's (a huge Star Trek fan) voice, the doctors called this accidental or without purpose, but I knew otherwise.

- The long, long wait for her eyes to open or for her to begin speaking.
- Staff entering a room without knocking, to empty trash, etc. A parent becomes afraid to leave a child at all. I luckily could afford around the clock support, never leaving Kelly alone in a room. The fear of molestation was present always, because a child cannot protest while in coma.
- Meeting people whose children never came out of coma, or who did, but couldn't be expected to live normally
- Driving a car even briefly. A person fears that as a caretaker, getting hurt or disabled would be devastating to the patient. Thus a mom like me is scared to leave her child at all, even to drive home for a shower.
- Facing rising expenses and pesky insurance persons. I'd tell any caretaker: "Get an attorney to take over your affairs at once, and avoid signing anything for a long, long time or until you know what future years may hold." I chose an attorney who did not work on commission, but this option isn't always available. And make sure you have a "rider" on your insurance for under or uninsured motorists!! Thanks to Jack Davis, we did.
- Fear of the nursing staff. I had a terrible tendency to exhaust myself doing everything for Kelly's wellbeing, but my conscience was clear. Naturally the nurses hated me. Several assured me she was not in pain because she wasn't crying—when I knew she was!
- I began to experience a fear of life. Can one endure living in a world where such horrible things like TBI happen? I wasn't sure for months about my own ability to live in the same world I once occupied innocently, unaware. Like a rape victim, I felt frightened everywhere, all of the time.
- Fear that I would run out of strength before nursing my child back to health. Part of me was already dead, but the rest of me needed to stay alive. My job was not yet finished.

What mixed feelings we all had the last day in Brenner's. We were released from the hospital in Winston-Salem only to be re-consigned to another, less familiar one. But we were not moving backwards. The only uplifting moment of that day was that Kelly's high school principal came to send her off, promising her that when she came back to high school, "Whatever you need, it's yours!" He hugged Kelly as she was assisted into our car, and we left home.

The Land In-Between

> Life is richest when we realize that we are all snowflakes. Each of us is absolutely beautiful and unique. And we are here for a very short time.
>
> – Elisabeth Kübler-Ross

When you enter a rehabilitation unit for the traumatically brain injured, you enter a place Kelly and I call "The Land In Between." A number of patients, quite simply, are neither dead nor alive. They have come to rehab because their brains do not allow them to function in life as they knew it. Although some are recovering well, many are only alive because of modern mechanized medicine. Some are learning to speak or walk; others to communicate through voice boards. Some have nowhere else to go, for their families are not equipped to deal with a person neither dead nor alive and functioning normally. Many families at Myers Lake Rehab show the same numb expressions. They are learning how to grieve for the living.

In life and literature, death always seems to be one's ultimate fear. This is fallacy. The Land In Between is the ultimate fear, and dying can be the mercy of God. In rehab, Kelly and I learned not to be afraid of dying, for living through trauma is scary enough.

Leaving this land is the goal, the only goal. You do not leave it just by being discharged and going home. You leave by sweat and tears and faith, by physical torture (therapy), by refusal to stay. You leave by remembering the Elephant Man.

The Elephant Man

The elephant man started as a voice in the night. Kelly was frightened by the high-pitched wailing of elephants, and a relentless cry of some unknown patient down the hall resembled this. I slept on a pallet by her bed, and we would hold hands and try to sleep as he screamed and screamed. During the days, the cry began to sound funny; we would laugh each time it began. Sometimes the only two choices are to laugh or weep, and humor is definitely the healthier option for convalescents.

We were both convalescents, my daughter and I—she from her brain injury, I from my terrors that we would never leave this place. We tried to laugh and the humor was black. If a patient beat his head on the wall, we laughed. If Elephant Man shrieked, we cackled and made jokes. It was nearly Halloween, and Kelly wanted to unlock all the patients' doors on October 31st to cause havoc and to finally get a glimpse of the elephants. This humor kept us sane, and only left me when I saw the parents of those who would obviously never leave. How can we adapt to this hollow way of living, this half-life? I began to wonder what the Elephant Man's mother was like. How could she have the strength to endure? Would she herself commit suicide? I was almost suicidal, and my child was improving.

In Kelly's third week of in-patient rehab, we went a little early to the enormous Physical Therapy (PT) room for her to lift weights. Perhaps sixty people were already there, hard at work. As my child lay prostrate, holding a weight bar aloft, I heard the elephant wail softly. Kelly was concentrating and didn't hear. While Susie, the young therapist, worked with Kelly, I wandered toward the sound. He was sitting alone in a wheelchair, and the sight of him astounded me. I had always imagined an elderly stroke victim in my mind's eye; yet here was a boy of perhaps twenty, drooling and staring mindlessly at the ceiling. He was strapped safely in his chair, waiting. Waiting and alone. Young, blonde, blue-eyed, wasted, a permanent resident of this land. At that moment, I knew Kelly would leave, for such an existence is only possible for those stronger than we are.

(Now, years later, Kelly has the usual problems of work, relationships, and parenting. I have the housewife blues. During our whiny times, one of us will turn to the other and say, "Remember the Elephant Man." Complaints cease.)

The Dam-Man

I met the Dam-Man on my second day at Myers Lake Rehab, and the sight of him made me want to cry; yet his actions made me laugh. He was in casts from head to toe and being rolled about on a sort of bed/ chair combination that accommodated his numerous broken limbs. He was probably about 35 years old, judging from the fact that his mother looked about fifty going on a hundred. This wizened old woman rolled the Dam-Man outdoors to the courtyard several times a day to smoke. She had varicose veins and looked arthritic. I finally had the nerve to join them for a quick "stress" cigarette—the wicked weed I had "quit" in August 1992. Now it was the only thing available to me to calm my nerves.

"I'm waiting for my daughter Kelly to finish physical therapy," I began. "How long have you been here?"

The Dam-Man mumbled from the bandages, "Over a month now, and it makes me so damn mad that I can't smoke in my room! I was working construction on a dam, lost my balance and fell 80 feet onto a concrete slab. I hurt everywhere and I can't even smoke until Mom can roll me out here. I'm scared she'll hurt herself as I make her come so often. We come about six times a day. Whenever I can!"

Just then a physical therapist came and pushed the Dam-Man away for some newly devised form of physical torture, and his mother approached me, glad to have a conversation-mate.

"My oldest boy died two years ago in a car wreck," she announced bluntly, "and I'll do anything to see this boy gets well. His brains ain't messed up much, but the rest of him is pretty awful. We won't know about his walkin' for a long time yet, so I'll just see you a lot, I guess. Your little girl messed up?"

I explained that Kelly had injured only her head in an accident, but that she was relearning how to walk and talk. The Dam-Man's mother was jealous when she heard me say "walk," but she smiled and went on.

"He don't have much future for working," she declared, "and he just lives for these times he can sneak a cigarette. The nurses won't bring him out here. It hurts me, but it's all he looks forward to anymore."

"I know." I lit my fourth of the morning.

Thinking back on the Dam-Man, I realize the value of short-term goals, especially when you're scared to make any long-term goals. In rehab, long-term anything for the critically injured is an unknown. Few doctors in this litigious world will predict a long-term outcome. Thus, short-term becomes the grail. A cigarette for him and me, a few steps and words for Kelly.

"That man looks like a mummy. I don't like him," said Kelly when we passed the Dam-Man in the hallway. Kelly's only emotion at that time was anger. Generally, she was rather emotionless.

Mike from Charlotte

Some people can change your life in just a few moments, and Mike was one of them for Kelly and me. He was 26 years old, had a head full of dark wavy hair, and a wide smile that was a permanent fixture on his face. After the scores of patients with TBI, who stared blankly around the spacious walls of the PT room, his alert gaze was incongruous, even shocking.

It had been a bad day for Kelly. Still seeing double (diplopia), the therapist had again forgotten to bring her an eye patch (you only see double when using two eyes). Kelly had swum laps already, had a grueling speech therapy session, and lifted weights to the point of exhaustion. When Mike entered our world, she was reclined on a mat, lifting a barbell above her head to build arm strength while attempting to memorize "We hold our truths to be self-evident" (doctor's orders). There was no light in Kelly's blue eyes, but I did smile when the doctor asked her to recite the Preamble to the Constitution and he started by saying "We hold these truths..." My daughter stopped him and said, "We hold these truths... comes from the Declaration of Independence!" And she was right.

Susie, the PT, came and told Kelly she was going to walk a few steps that day, with no aids. Kelly often used her wheelchair back as a walker. My child politely declined with a nod. Suddenly one of the patients, Mike, approached in a wheelchair at high speed, screeched to a halt, and said, "Walk for me, Kelly!" She glanced at his handsome smile, and the light went on for a moment. "I don't think so," she said, smiling back.

"But I want to see you do it," Mike said with an enticing grin.

"What are you doing here?" she whispered candidly. In-patients at Myers Lake Rehab rarely used tact when discussing their injuries. "How can you smile in this place?"

Without hesitation, he told her.

"I was coming out of my condo one night at about 9 p.m., and a man was crouched beside my car. He had just robbed a bank. I guess he thought I was a policeman coming after him, because he jumped up and shoved a knife in my back, then started running. Now I can't walk anymore; my spinal cord was severed. I'm here learning to handle the wheelchair better. Hey, want to see me do a wheelie?" He demonstrated while Susie waited patiently.

Kelly pondered. "What do you have to smile about?" she asked again, echoing my own thoughts.

Mike wheeled up close to her face which still rested on the mat.

"God took care of me," he said calmly. "I have the most beautiful wife in the world, and a three-year-old daughter at home waiting to hug me when I get out of here. God let me have them before my attack, and I can still work at my job from a wheelchair. So, I have a child to carry my name and love me, a job, and a perfect wife. Most people here don't even have a mind. So, Kelly Bouldin, get up and walk for me since I can't."

Sweat dripping from her forehead, Kelly wobbled to an erect position, reached for the handles of her chair, and pulled upward. Turning first to me, then Susie, then Mike, she began to walk toward Susie's open arms. She took at least 14 steps before grasping for support, turned to Mike, and beamed.

"I'll see you tomorrow," he grinned. "Keep it up," he called as he did another terrific wheelie and sped away. I found myself wishing Kelly's spine had been injured instead of her brain. Somehow I'd missed the fact that Myers Lake Rehab not only worked with patients suffering from TBI, but also those with spinal injuries.

I began to notice that most patients gave praise with their eyes and actions. Somehow words had no meaning for them. A look said everything.

(At home, months later, when Kelly's friends came over with problems like *Oh, my life is awful... I'm grounded for two weeks...*, Kelly and I exchange a wordless glance. We think of Mike, who, like my child, knows what a problem is. Such adolescent concerns used to anger us both, but we've learned to accept them. They are indeed problems for those who haven't experienced worse. Mike, we wonder how you are now. You gave us the gift of perspective, and we think of you whenever Kelly has to confront a "problem.")

Paradox

I was terrified to learn that Kelly's post-wreck IQ was in the cellar until I was told doctors couldn't assess her IQ accurately, yet. Kelly couldn't write rapidly enough with her hand impairment to complete a timed IQ test. I asked to see some questions presented to her verbally. One was "What would you do if you were running late to meet friends at a movie?" Kelly responded: "Miss the movie!" Well, she didn't get a point for that; the correct answer was "hurry." Kelly missed several similar questions, even though her responses seemed to make sense to me. What's more, her answers all fit with what I know of my rather sardonic daughter. Also, I looked at her analysis of a "wise saying" or two. Kelly had to make sense of the phrase: "People in glass houses shouldn't throw stones." I felt sure that my child had never heard that saying before, and that made me wonder: why not ask a teenager why "you can check out any time you like, but you can never leave..."? She'd know the verse was referring to addiction in the song "Hotel California." I think the adages on neuropsychological tests are archaic and could use a little refreshing.

Victoria's Secret

My cousin Emily Anderson came to visit Kelly yesterday, bringing a lovely gift from Victoria's Secret. Emily is in her late 20s and works in Charlotte. She has long golden hair and a smile like Christmas morning. From the moment she entered the room, the oppressive atmosphere of "hospital" lifted. Kelly reached for her package and with help from Emily, revealed a precious little nightgown. Kelly beamed. "I like it," she said.

I was stunned, and in seconds, I was laughing. This gift was not what I was expecting. I had become used to gifts like marking pens and flip-erase pads. What I loved most about this gift was that it came with a host of positive implications. This was the kind of gift a normal teenaged girl might like. Did Emily think Kelly would be normal again? Emily began chatting with Kelly, whose animated face was not the face of an hour ago in therapy. I saw no pain, no fear in her face. Emily was asking her advice, as if her advice mattered.

"See, I'm dating this guy I really like, but I don't adore his family. And I'm scared and confused. He gave me a diamond, and I'm nearly thirty, and this may be my last chance at marriage. But I'm just not sure."

Kelly reached over to Emily who was sitting on the foot of her bed. Kelly whispered, "Keep the ring, ditch the guy." And I laughed because the advice was so astute, and because Kelly had given me the little gift of humor without even knowing how funny she was.

The next day, my sister Clara (whom I call LaLa) came to spend the night with us because she knew I was nearing breakdown levels. Two things happened that neither of us will ever forget. My sister is a divorced single mom, whose son had given her an air mattress to use in his small apartment. Marc had shown her how to inflate the plastic blob without a pump, and we sat on the floor to blow. But we found no tiny plastic holes to blow into. We draped it on Kelly's bed and she helped us look, moving the vast tent of folds around the bed. Finally Kelly found an arm.

"It's a *raincoat*," she said, looking at us as if we were imbeciles. And it was. At that point, Kelly was smarter than we were, and LaLa and I collapsed in laughter. We still can't look at a plastic raincoat without remembering and cracking up.

The next day, Kelly showed LaLa the small cafeteria where patients were supposed to eat their meals. Kelly often called nurses to bring her food on a tray, for she didn't like the company of adult patients in rehab. But that day was for showing off. Kelly used a walker to steer us into the line, and then asked me to take her walker away. She leaned on the cafeteria rails for support, and with shaking hands, gathered her own lunch without assistance. LaLa and I watched her do this seemingly simple task. We sat down and just watched her. LaLa looked at me and our gaze held. Without using words, she was saying, "This is not the same child that left Winston-Salem. This girl's going to be all right. She can do things on her own." Epiphany. We wouldn't be in our dark place forever. TBI would not defeat Kelly.

Leaving / Fleeing Rehab

If I ever let Kelly down during her entire recovery, it was my decision to leave rehab after less than a month. Stories were filtering back to me from parents who had also left earlier than doctors recommended, so I knew this was a possibility. I was, to put it mildly, "losing it!" I had decided early on to experience what my child was experiencing, in order to understand her state of mind. No outside trips to the hairdresser for me. I stayed by her side every moment. I watched as other moms left during therapy sessions to enjoy a bit of shopping. Space aliens couldn't have affected me more strangely. I sat in on 8–10 hours a day of grueling speech, occupational, recreational, and physical therapy sessions. I even attended her counseling sessions when I was allowed. How else could I learn what to do when Kelly came home? Most of the therapists willingly allowed me in their rooms, and some shut me out in the hall, but Kelly knew I was in earshot most of the time.

Small things began driving us crazy—no vanilla Dixie cups like they had at Brenner's hospital, no privacy, no quiet, numerous cussing scary people in her group therapy sessions, a huge and intimidating neuropsychologist named Lynn, and worst of all, only one other teenager—

Christy, from Winston-Salem. This child had motioned to me once from her wheelchair, and I bent near her bandaged face.

"They bathe me in cold water," she whispered. Her mother was not with her then, so I exploded to nearby staff. (Since that time, after protests from me and her mom and others, patients in this rehab center have been age-grouped, but Kelly was with severely injured adults who frightened her always.)

One midnight, I took a shower and returned to find a male orderly just standing and staring at my sleeping child. At that moment, I had had enough. My husband said, "We're leaving. You're all falling apart. Kelly can walk some now and we're going home!"

Dr. McWhorter and Dr. David Kelly of WFU/BMC concurred, and the Martinat Center of Forsyth Hospital[2] in Winston-Salem agreed to see Kelly for outpatient therapy daily (stretching their three-visits-per-week rule). Dr. McDonald was quite unhappy with me, however. He begged me to keep Kelly there two more weeks at least, warning that her behavior was still "socially unacceptable" for the return home. I didn't appreciate then what he meant. I wanted us home!

It was explained to me that one reason Kelly was sent to Charlotte for in-patient rehabilitation was to withdraw from all medications while under constant doctor's watch. I'd like to have known that sooner, as the ordeal would have been easier. In hindsight, this was a good thing. One day at Myers Lake Rehab, Kelly had panicked, thinking she was swallowing her tongue. Dr. McDonald appeared in minutes to explain to her that the left side of her mouth was still more paralyzed than her right, and the sensation was normal. So Kelly left this facility on no medications and without too much fear of seizure. She had developed an allergy to the anti-seizure medicine Dilantin, but that had been carefully withdrawn. Ironically, doctors refused to prescribe pain medication for Kelly's head and muscle aches. One said, "Nicotine is the only safe drug for her at present, and she can quit later." Evidently, even anti-depressants were not safe for Kelly, whose brain might overreact to them. Thus going home was scary and yet wonderful, the first huge step toward normalcy in her life and ours.

During the car ride home, Kelly whispered to me, "I kept my promise to Dad. I said I would leave Myers Lake Rehab walking, not in a wheelchair. And that's what I did!"

---

[2] This wonderful institution is now called the Novant Health Martinat Outpatient Rehabilitation Center.

We were both so happy to come home. We had no way of knowing that our most difficult trials were just beginning. Dante was right, for hell has many levels. And it's a long way back from the darkness. Despite all Kelly learned and relearned in rehab, we hated being locked up. In rehabilitation centers for patients with severe TBI, "lock and key" may keep one safe from other patients, but the jail-like atmosphere was frightening and, at times, suffocating.

4 Socially Inappropriate Behavior

As said before, my husband and I were not adequately prepared for Kelly's return home. The transition from inpatient rehab to home and outpatient therapy was complex, difficult. Once the immediate joy of being home after what seemed like an eternity faded, the doctors' warnings of "socially unacceptable/inappropriate behavior" from Kelly began to take shape.

In retrospect, the problems arose mainly from Kelly's very literal interpretations of words and events. If I said I was blue, she said I looked pink to her. If she heard the word "birthday," she wanted presents, even if the birthday wasn't hers.

She had no tact. If a friend placed a foot on Kelly's bed, she responded, "Get if off!" She could have simply asked politely for its removal.

She often revealed the secrets of her friends. For instance, she asked a friend if she was still driving illegally—in front of the friend's mother. What Kelly wanted to know about, she would ask, regardless of the appropriate time, place, and person.

Little mannerisms popped up out of place. Kelly would straighten a bra strap in mixed company, for instance. My daughter was quick to inform friends when they were "boring." She also asked them to leave if she was tired of their company. Basically, she made friends extremely uncomfortable because they didn't know what she might say or do next.

Yet much of the time, Kelly was very sweet and loving. She expressed her feelings openly, voicing likes and dislikes clearly. To those of us who loved her best, much of this activity was humorous. However, the very remarks that made friend Zach laugh out loud, made friend Carla leave quickly with tears about to fall.

What we were all dealing with was a fifteen-year-old body and the mind of a kindergartener or toddler. Because Kelly acted her age at times, we didn't realize she was basically still a child acting maturely, not the opposite.

I should have better prepared Kelly's friends for her socially inappropriate behavior, but how could I? I had no idea, aside from what others had warned me about, what to say about how my child might act. In hindsight, I should have merely lied and told them all that Kelly would be back to her old self again in a year or two. Hearing this, her friends might have coped better; however, I chose honesty and simply tried to prepare visitors for Kelly's erratic behavior. Someone should have warned me of what returning home with obvious disabilities would mean for Kelly. Perhaps they did and I wasn't ready to listen.

Soon, many of Kelly's friends stopped visiting (after about six weeks) and she fell into a depression, cushioned only by her inability to realize the full implications of her abandonment. Now where should Kelly and I look for hope? What doctor would feel free to encourage us? Who would be willing to state that my daughter's mind would indeed recover?

(I want to tell others that this can happen, and you can dare to hope. There are things you can do to enhance your odds of a full recovery. You just have to discover them. Pre-Internet, I was handicapped by lack of knowledge. Much has changed since '92.)

Home from Myers Lake Rehab - November 1992

I'm glad Kelly made me buy a daybed last year with a trundle underneath. I can sleep in the trundle right beside her so that she can't get out of bed in the night and try walking to the bathroom (and probably fall) without stepping on my head. She resists having me steady her as she walks, but her gait is so unsteady and her vision seems to be completely double.

It's ironic, but a big problem we're having is exactly the same thing that gave us much joy in the hospital. Kelly is giving too many orders. We were glad to hear her speak any words at all just a few weeks ago, and in the hospital, it seemed normal for her to say, "Get me a Coke," or "Bring me that brush." At home, it is beginning to sound rude; but we've trained her to issue commands. We've been waiting on her hand and foot for so long. This process of "aging up" is going to take a while.

I'm trying to tell her that "I will do anything for you that you can't do for yourself, but you're going to have to do the other things." I am raising Kelly for the second time!

Dr. McWhorter warned me: "You will be her best friend, or her worst enemy." I realized that she must learn to do things for herself now.

Earlier today, Mike Sellars came over, and was gingerly trying to figure Kelly out. Her commands puzzled him, but he waited on her and wasn't complaining. He looked so sad. I guess he expected her to be all well the minute she reentered our home. Like all of us, he wants to fix her right now, not wanting to accept that we must all be patient! Mike is nursing a possum back to health for the Humane Society. I think he will try to do the same here, but his patience is going to run out.

Today was both funny and sad. Kelly stumbled into the kitchen and told me she was going on a walk, even though it was raining and she stumbled badly when walking unassisted. I'm guessing she wanted to smoke a cigarette, because her last visitors had been smoking out on the porch. I thought for a moment and told her we'd have to have more liberal rules around here. I chose to let her smoke with friends on the porch, since it wasn't safe for her to hide it. She couldn't drink or smoke marijuana, so I'd have to let her be "bad" somehow. She had to be a teenager. I sometimes wished a doctor in rehab hadn't told me that nicotine would be the only safe drug for my child, which I had idiotically told her. There'd been no secrets between us within the confines of Myers Lake Rehab. I was feeling very tired. I hadn't realized how hard coming home would be. This year's Christmas wouldn't be very merry.

Kelly told me she was worried about the dark hair appearing on her face due to the steroid medication she'd taken. A little Sally Hansen will take care of the lip, but more importantly, I suddenly realized that Kelly was beginning to notice small things. The downside to this was that I hoped we could fix things as fast as she noticed them. I saw this as another one of the many hats I would be asked to wear. Mother "The Fixer!" I'm also going to dye her hair blonde again very soon. It turned quite dark in the hospitals, as we rarely paid the sun a visit. Her face had become rather pale and puffy as well. On the bright side, Kelly was now off all medications; however, she thought she was ugly now. I wish she knew how lovely she looked even with her problems. Occasionally, when a friend was around, the light went back on full force in her eyes. She sparkled again and my heart seemed to sparkle

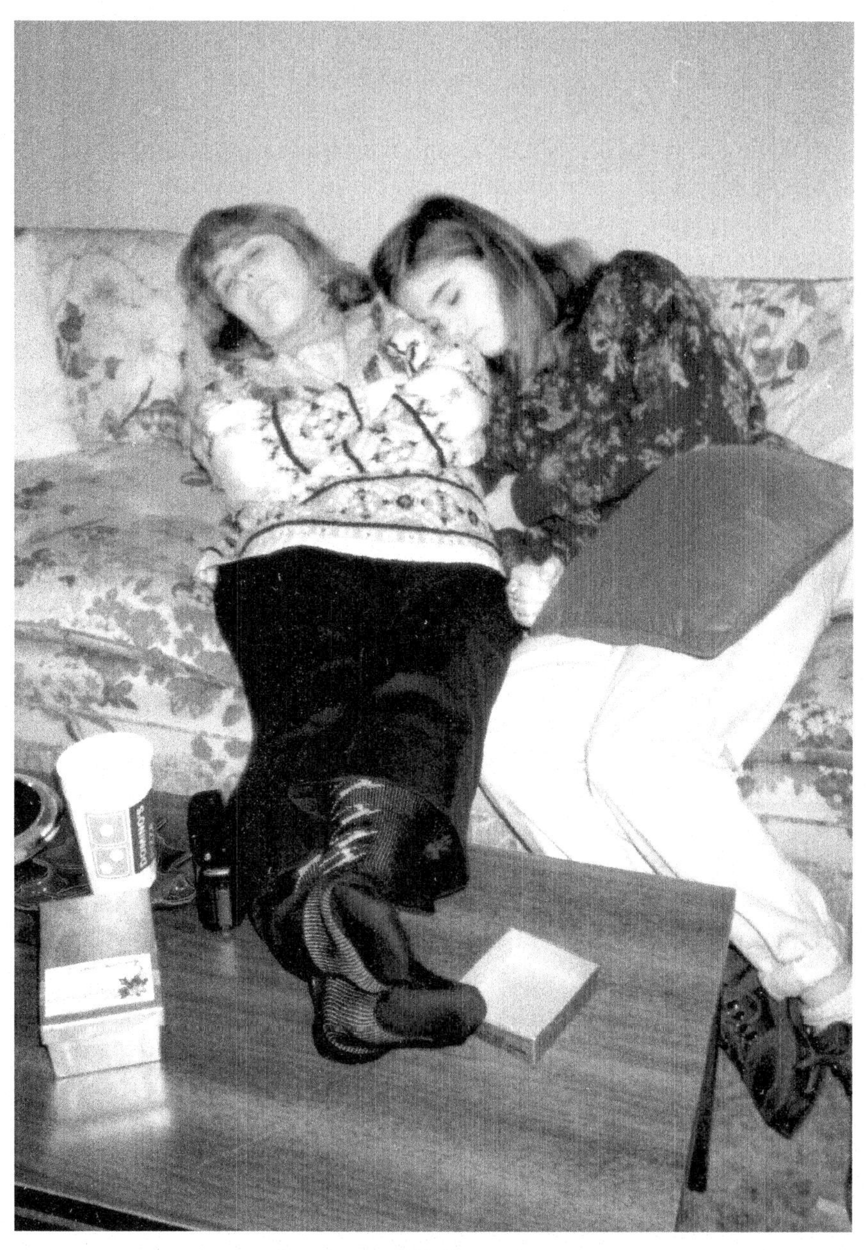

Carolyn and Kelly on the sofa

with her. I was living for those moments. If they could come once, they would return more and more again.

Kelly's clothes were too tight around the waist. That area seemed sort of frozen and a bit swollen. She got so mad when I said we'd have to cut back on junk food.

"I haven't gained any weight!" she screamed at me, and then called me, "a fucking bitch!" I knew it was easier for her to swallow ice cream. I also knew she avoided cutting meat, and preferred holding a chicken sandwich left-handed. She didn't want kids noticing her rather severe hand tremors. I'd have to prepare healthier foods that are easy to swallow, and cut things up for a while. Would this be another hat for me to wear? That night, I let out her cheerleader uniforms as much as I could. She thought I shrank them. This was all too painful for me to endure.

Kelly was in denial, but I guess she couldn't cope any other way. She seemed devoid of tact, and she had once been so clever with words and people. Either her tact had not yet returned, or she was just too weary to try remembering it. I am scared, though, because doctors have said she may have a lifelong problem maintaining relationships. However, this mother can't be discouraged that easily. I will remain the "F.B." (Fucking Bitch) until I manage to teach my daughter some form of manners, I hope.

She told me she hates being sick. I said, "You're not sick... you're broken! You call me F.B. and I'll call you B.D.—my broken daughter... bad daughter... beautiful and brave daughter!"

(I still call her B.D.)

Other Wardrobe Malfunctions - December '92

There was one part of amnesia that surprised me totally. Kelly didn't remember how to dress appropriately. She would put on jeans and a sweater, which was fine and very appropriate for winter wear; but then she would put on "summer" sandals, and they didn't even match each other. She once put on mismatched socks, but I thought it was an accident due to poor eyesight. She continued trying to dress herself, but at least one part of each outfit looked wrong. My child didn't know how to do the "fashion thing" anymore, and she was once so very good at it.

I began to realize that she was putting on the first thing she grabbed from her drawer or closet, without trying to match colors or styles. Mainly, I realized that she never checked the back of her closet for forgotten attire, or separated summer from winter clothing. I then decided to take an hour, when Kelly's friends had her busy, and take all of her summer clothing to the attic. I also took all of the sandals. Then I put matching outfits together. Just a few of them right in front. Problem solved.

To Be Or Not To Be

Kelly's first post-TBI Christmas, gloomy in itself, was over. She'd barely glanced at her numerous gifts. We were home from visiting relatives by Saturday afternoon, and no one came to visit. Kelly waited by the telephone all day, the silence only broken by a much-needed review of math facts, multiplication, and division. She went to bed early, and I lay in the trundle beside her, wondering again how to help her socially. On Sunday morning, she stayed in bed late. I went for coffee before looking back in her downstairs bedroom.

"I should have died on September 17th," she muttered, turning away from me. I told her not to say that again. Then Kelly got up and threw a textbook into her full-length mirror, smashing it. "I'm going out," she said in her nightclothes, and I blocked her path to the door. After a sad, brief wrestling match, we both landed on the bed. She shook, unable to cry, but I was crying. "You look funny when you cry," she said, trying to attack me and thus the rest of the world verbally.

"Call your friends!" I ordered.

"No, they *don't care*," she responded.

"They care, but they don't read minds!" I answered. "They may think you're busy studying or doing your exercises." I put the telephone in her hands and left the room. Soon I could hear the slow sounds of her voice, and a receiver smashing down. I returned to her, and she said, "I called Carla and told her I was lonely. She said she was sleeping and to call back later. I was right. *No one cares*."

"I meant call your real friends. The ones from Summit School you've known 15 years!" Exiting the room again, I left Kelly with phone in hand. My child had made a group of attractive, new, young people in the months prior to her wreck, girls on her cheerleading squad, and boys in her Honors classes. The Reynolds cheerleaders had met in the spring of 8th grade while trying out for the public high school squad. Over the summer, some of them had come by daily, called incessantly, and placed Kelly at the pinnacle of new popularity. Most of these "friends" disappeared, however, when Kelly returned from rehab still quite ill and not like her former self. At least the girls did. Many boys continued to check in on her. Interestingly, they seemed to care less about appearances. At any rate, I allowed a half hour to pass, wondering if Kelly was dismantling her room, or talking on the phone.

Then she called out to me, "I called Nicole. She'll be here soon." My daughter was smiling widely for the first time since her 15th birthday. In about twenty minutes, our doorbell rang, and five young females trooped into the house. Nicole, best Summit friend since age two, had called other old buddies, and there they were hugging Kelly, telling them how they missed her and never knew when to come over—basically, just loving her. This moment was perhaps the greatest turning point in Kelly's recovery, because she learned two things: she still had friends who would help her recover, and she had a measure of control back. Raised to be self-reliant, she had to learn to ask others for help and to lean on them for support.

Nicole Price was Kelly's friend who broke an arm playing Wonder Woman at age two; who played Breyer Horses with Kelly at age seven; who double-dated with Kelly to her first ballroom dancing cotillion at age 13. She went trick-or-treating with Kelly each year, and played on her field hockey team in junior high. Nicole went to camps with Kelly, Camp Thunderbird and Camp Cheerio. No other friend was in a better position to help my child, to help her remember events from a forgotten past. Along with Suzanne Davis, another constant childhood playmate, Nicole began driving Kelly to school events. Suzanne took her to the beach, and often included her in parties in her home. They helped save Kelly's sanity while doctors were saving her life. Bless them. Some things she will never forget—nor will I.

Mood Swings - January '93

One day Kelly said to me, "I'm tired of living under a microscope." She rightly felt that friends and teachers examined every little thing she did. Well, I did that also, looking for signs of improvement, of a plateau that never really happened (thank God), watching for any small signal alerting us to her needs. I started to cry a bit that day, and Kelly came to me and said, "You have to allow me a bad mood once in a while. I'm okay, but you get depressed if I'm even a little bit sad... can you stop that?" I realized how profoundly she was analyzing her own recovery, and how dangerously intertwined she and I had become. We lived and worked too close in proximity.

Back To School Part-Time: Early - '93

I never chose my battles,
I have a broken wing,
But I can sound the battle cry
For those who cannot sing.

– Nathalia Crane, "The Colors"

All of our doctors told us to place Kelly back into her most familiar environment, into a school that was so familiar that her memories would "trigger back" instantaneously. But she had only been at Reynolds High School for about three weeks. Would this be familiar enough to help her remember the details of her life? We came home from Myers Lake Rehab in late November 1992, and knew Kelly could only attend classes, with assistance, for an hour or two a day. We'd begin after Christmas. She would need time to continue her rehabilitation, to relearn to walk, talk, write, and so forth. She still had double vision, suffered from extreme fatigue, and couldn't remember most of what occurred from one hour to the next.

Ultimately I met with guidance at the high school, and after a great deal of begging, the school agreed to allow Kelly to re-enter on a special basis. I would handle make up work for the first semester (because I was a licensed secondary teacher in North Carolina), and a homebound teacher would work with her for the second semester. If she attended classes, I had to remain somewhere in the building. I'd been told Kelly was the high school's first TBI-certified student; therefore this seemed reasonable.

So I spent most days in the teachers' lounge. The high school was undergoing renovations at the time, and this three-story building no longer had banisters. Would a limping child who could barely walk a straight line or see with any clarity be able to handle this? Well, there was only one way to find out. Mornings at school, then homebound instruction, then therapy, then sleep, and repeat.

The Gift

Mrs. Gibson was a wonderful homebound teacher who, miraculously, had experienced students with TBI in the past. In the spring of 1993, she started working with Kelly. She was patient and would always allow Kelly to rest her head on the dining room table when she couldn't keep her eyes open.

Somehow Mrs. Gibson managed to drill history and science facts into Kelly anyway. She would put Kelly's work on poster paper in large letters, which helped her see, and she provided a study guide for data. I copied Mrs. Gibson's methods to complete first semester assignments, working in stolen minutes, like suppertime and midnight.

Whenever she felt Kelly had mastered a unit, Mrs. Gibson tested her immediately on it. She usually used oral methods or short-answer format in large print. She taught me so much about helping a child with double vision who couldn't hold a pen well or retain facts more than an hour or two. I owe this woman much. Mr. Mock at the high school was right in saying, "Take this gift (homebound instruction). It will help Kelly more than you know!"

The IEP

I shudder to approach this area. An Individualized Education Program (IEP) is essential (but tedious) to any student returning to school after a severe head injury. Such documentation, required by law to equalize educational opportunities for the disabled, can be a huge blessing; however, even a former teacher like me, somewhat acquainted with disability law, can be dismayed by the process. I was overwhelmed and completely unprepared. I saw the process as a blur. Parents are called in to meet with the on-site person in charge of special needs for students—also with the principal, guidance counselor, classroom teachers, and an official from the central school office, who may meet you only once or twice. You are asked to elucidate whatever needs your child has... large print books? Extended time for tests? *et cetera!* The problem is, until your child is actually in school, you have no real concept of his or her needs so you end up signing this document rather blindly, having listened to the "experts" in a school, who also know little about TBI. This vital, life-giving, terribly meaningful document can be signed by the unsuspecting parent who is in too much shock to realize its importance.

Someone will tell you to call a conference to alter your IEP if new needs arise, but you will forget this because you are busy nursing your child. So you will live with both kindness and random injustices from the school because you are unaware of his/her rights under IDEA—Individuals with Disabilities Education Act—a pamphlet someone handed you in the ICU and you dumped in the hospital trash without reading.

After a while, you will begin to learn the politics of your particular school system. You will learn (as I did) that if you want an IEP changed, the only way is to request a new conference. But your child's needs may be urgent, and your request may take weeks. I found myself weeping one day because Kelly needed *word banks* ("optional answers" list) for tests, and teachers were not providing them because this need was not specifically written in Kelly's IEP. Somehow I'd believed all teachers would accommodate her needs spontaneously, and I'm sure that some did. However, Kelly's inability to recall a word without visual options needed immediate attention. So I consulted a professional friend, Mr. Jim Bray, founder of the North Carolina Governor's School.

Jim said, "The next time someone delays an IEP meeting, start your conversations with these words: 'Before I litigate'..." This surprising but firm advice worked, although I alienated administrators who saw my demeanor change overnight. A dawning realization scared me to death—I knew more about TBI than most teachers did.

(By Kelly's fourth year in a public high school, we had the IEP right, but accomplishing this goal was a career in itself. I learned—and I repeat—if a need isn't specifically stated in an IEP, some teachers don't comply. Today this may be easier with computer programs, such as "Easy IEP.")

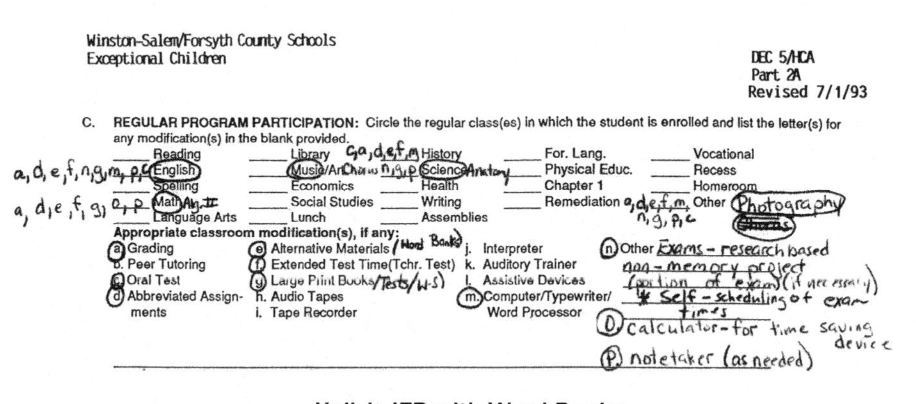

Winston-Salem/Forsyth County Schools
Exceptional Children

DEC 5/HCA
Part 2A
Revised 7/1/93

C. REGULAR PROGRAM PARTICIPATION: Circle the regular class(es) in which the student is enrolled and list the letter(s) for any modification(s) in the blank provided.

____ Reading	____ Library	a, d, e, f, m History	____ For. Lang.	____ Vocational
a, d, e, f, n, g, m, p, c English	____ Music/Art Chorus	n, g, p Science Anatomy	____ Physical Educ.	____ Recess
____ Spelling	____ Economics	____ Health	____ Chapter 1	____ Homeroom
a, d, e, f, g, o, p Math Alg. II	____ Social Studies	____ Writing	____ Remediation	a, d, e, f, m, n, g, p, c Other Photography
____ Language Arts	____ Lunch	____ Assemblies		

Appropriate classroom modification(s), if any:

a. Grading	e. Alternative Materials (Word Banks)	j. Interpreter	n. Other Exams – research based non-memory project (portion of exam) (if necessary)
b. Peer Tutoring	f. Extended Test Time(Tchr. Test)	k. Auditory Trainer	* Self-scheduling of exam times
c. Oral Test	g. Large Print Books/Tests/W-S	l. Assistive Devices	o. calculator – for time saving device
d. Abbreviated Assignments	h. Audio Tapes	m. Computer/Typewriter/ Word Processor	p. notetaker (as needed)
	i. Tape Recorder		

Kelly's IEP with Word Banks

Downhill - 1/93

There was a fairly sizable snowstorm and a blanket of white covered most of the city. School was cancelled for that day, and a group of Kelly's old friends were going sledding on the hills of a nearby golf course. I discovered that Kelly was supposed to be included in this venture, until her friend Nora exclaimed, "Kelly will just slow us down!" So my child was left out—again. I appreciate the friend who told me this.

But even if Kelly had been asked, I couldn't have let her go, as she might have hit a tree or collided with a rock or something.

Kelly was a very unique fifteen-year-old when the accident happened. She wasn't finding herself. She already knew herself. She knew exactly who she was, which was an athlete, honors student, liked by all because she was a listener, and a leader. Most of all, she saw herself as an artist, dancer, equestrian, and cheerleader. These were the things she loved the most, what she felt good at and what she liked most about herself.

I remember talking to the mother of another child with TBI right after Kelly's car crash. I met her daughter, a teenaged girl who was smiling, but walking with a cane. I asked her, "What has been the hardest part of the last year for you?"

"The abandonment by friends," her mom interrupted. I had laughed and assured her that this would never be Kelly's problem, as her friends would never do that. But her friends were going on with their lives—doing sports she couldn't do, drinking beer she couldn't drink, driving cars she couldn't drive. Kelly would have loved to ride a horse, but doctors cautioned against this, saying "No horses, no skiing. You could hit your head again and another blow would be fatal."

What happens to a person who loves to be needed, when no one needs them anymore?

Raindrops - Early 1993

One very drizzly afternoon, Kelly looked out a window and said:

> When I was in a coma
> There was a terrible storm.
> For months
> It drizzled.
> Now I feel the raindrops
> Falling off the trees.

Only months from the wreck, I typed her exact words, and said, "You just wrote a poem."

She looked at the printed words and smiled.

"Why is it a poem?" she asked.

"It's a poem because you used a metaphor, which is a comparison of your wreck to a thunderstorm. One thing really means the other," I answered.

After that day, Kelly began to write more poetry, as this was something she could do when other kids were at school or socializing. She remembered the definition of metaphor, for most of her prior knowledge only needed a reminder to be called back. One of my treasures is Kelly's next poem (on page 61).

Kelly worked for a long time on this poem, typing on her old computer. She printed it out and gave it to me. "You're the shovel," she said. I will never receive a greater compliment. This was one of many little gifts she gave me every day. But I'm so afraid she'll be cutting down oak trees for a very long time.

The Meadow

I used to play in the meadow.
And I didn't notice
The weeds at my feet.
I could easily run
In the meadow.
I went into a forest
Far away from the meadow.
I had so far to travel
And the weeds
Were in my way.
But I had a shovel
To cut them with.
And I went on
Thinking this was easy.
Now I am deep in the forest
I still haven't reached the meadow.
The oaks are in my way.
but I am very near.
My hands and a
shovel
Are still my only tools.
I can see through the trees
The meadow is nearer
And seems so very far
So I hit them
With my shovel (this is impossible) and
I hit
And hit and
Hit them.
I will make them fall
And I know I will
Rest in
The meadow.

Two Semesters in One - Spring 1993

Physical therapists kept telling her one consistent thing: keep working until you drop. "You will experience your greatest improvements in the two years following your accident," said the doctors. The clock ran and Kelly worked. She managed to cry a few tears for the first time post-TBI.

Young friends kept telling her, "I miss the old Kelly. We had so much fun together!" She understood what they were saying, but refused to accept it. Why couldn't people accept what she was post-TBI, until she was once again the old Kelly to them? After all, there was only one Kelly and she was still healing. Only by studying hard could she possibly find the old Kelly, and it was all so very hard. Hour after hour, memorizing the same few words and dates. This repetition seemed endless.

Friends came by less often. Worse, some teachers didn't want to work with RJR's first TBI-certified student, feared it, or simply couldn't be bothered. I'd been given the home phone number of Kelly's teachers, but using them got us in trouble. When Kelly forgot her homework, I called the Spanish teacher:

"I'm cooking dinner. Why are you calling me at home? Can't she just copy her homework from the board?"

No, Kelly couldn't see it. And she couldn't write, either.

One day, after a morning at school, Kelly begged me to describe her personality. Wow, I thought. Can this be done in words? Kelly tells me she remembers, for instance, what having a best friend means. She recalls that, but she doesn't know how it *feels* to be a best friend. Amnesia, in Kelly's case, affected emotional memories more than mere facts or names.

Not the Cobra - Spring '93

I may not be able to explain a feeling or friendship, but I can write down something that her best friend did for her. As "The Follies," a fundraising talent show for Reynolds, approached, Kelly's junior varsity cheerleading squad was preparing a performance. The girls on the squad decided that they didn't want to perform without Kelly, who still walked very slowly and haltingly. Nicole then choreographed a dance with Kelly as a cobra rising from a grass basket and the other girls as harem dancers, performing around the swaying snake. All Kelly would have to do is rise up from the container and sway with the pulsing music. I was enchanted, thrilled that she could be included on a stage, and that the girls had not forgotten her.

However, Kelly surprised us all. "No, I can't be the cobra." She exclaimed. "Next year I will be on stage doing the dance. I won't go on stage and let people feel sorry for me."

Does this sound like sour grapes and ingratitude? I thought so at first, but then I realized that Kelly fully expected to be completely back to normal in several months. I was not going to be the one to squelch that particular dream. While she was fantasizing about dancing in one year, I was lying awake at night wondering how many other dreams might be smashed in the coming months.

However, Kelly's return to school was, as I've said, only part-time. Parents, teachers and advisors decided to focus on four core subjects: English, History, Spanish, and Science. If by a miracle she could catch up in these subjects, she would be considered a sophomore in the fall of 1993, and meet her goal. She also had to complete her P.E. requirement—somehow!

Kelly would ask, "Promise me I can stay with my class. Promise me that!" This I promised, wisely or not.

Kelly's greatest joy this winter was donning her cheerleading black-and-gold costume and sitting in the bleachers with her '92-'93 squad. During basketball season, the squad sat on the lowest bleacher, so climbing wasn't necessary, and most cheers were only hand movements. All the girls helped Kelly relearn a few chants and clapping motions. She was sad not to dance at half time, but overjoyed just to be with her peers in uniform. This was "normal" teenager stuff for my baby girl, but I was afraid it would all end soon.

The Curse of Cheerleading

In the late spring of 1993, Kelly, formerly one of the best cheerleaders/choreographers on her squad, did not make the team for '93-'94. Yes, she was still unstable, but her friends wanted her back. They spent days teaching Kelly enough moves to qualify. I don't know why we were all hopeful.

I was secretly told that two of the "cheer moms" complained to the principal and others about having a student with traumatic brain injury on the squad. Kelly might collapse and hurt their daughters in a pyramid or something.

It was rumored that the cheerleading faculty advisor cast a negative vote for Kelly. I guess there was just too much liability and responsibility involved in a handicapped person being a member of a cheerleading squad. This was after I offered to sign all liability release forms, not that anything I did would have made a difference.

In the fall of 1993, another try-out was held for the next basketball season, and Kelly was faced with more disappointment. A request to merely practice with the girls was denied.

I couldn't help but realize how wonderful it was to have academic help for our daughter. Bob and I just wished the administration cared a little more about the mental and physical health of someone who was injured. The school gave her a great deal, but had—albeit without menace—taken away her sense of self, her plan for recovery and her means of social re-entry. No more cheer practices. We were not equipped to witness this death of compassion.

My Kelly needed an identity badly. She had been an artist, and now couldn't participate due to her hand impairment and tremors. Once an equestrian, she could no longer risk riding horses. She was no longer allowed to cheer or to attend a single cheerleading practice after her freshman year.

On a napkin I wrote, "Red tape. A good color. Bloody and deadly. I really wish Kelly were involved in a sport with a different image (not cheerleading). I do not wish Kelly to cheer for personal popularity and glory. I wish her to re-learn the musculature of her body."

I also wanted her to be socially "on the map" of her school. She needed rides to games, friends to sit with, and so on. Oh, well. The red tape continued to roll from the Bouldins to the school system and back again.

Soon after the abortive cheer tryouts, a close friend asked Kelly to describe how things at school were going. She didn't answer at that moment, but later scribbled:

> Here is who I am. A boy I liked is gone now. I was embarrassing. Girlfriends forget you, too. I am never around when plans are made. Teachers forget word banks. Come at 6th period to make up the test. No, go to study hall and complete it there. Complete another teacher's paper too, but only after chorus rehearsals. Get your service hours done. Report to the office. Who am I? Where am I?

I was encouraging Kelly to write for therapy while she was deciding which hand shook the least. Seems like we both had more questions than answers.

Frustration - Early '93

Doctor McDonald at Myers Lake Rehab had explained to me the dangers of allowing Kelly to sleep as much as she wanted to. Such a paradox: she is wounded, weary, but must stay awake for her brain to come alive. Last night I went into our unfinished basement to hide from the world. I scribbled this really bad poem to give her one day. I felt ambivalent about waking my exhausted child to do one more homework assignment.

Backward Time (for Kelly)

I tell you this in cryptic rhyme
This time for us is backward time.
The wounded body cannot heal
By resting. Likewise, just to feel
That tears again can fall and spread
You must be numb and inward dead,
For then when ice surrounds the heart
You feel the hottest tears depart
And sleep, the enemy, would come
You banish it, for to succumb
Is deadly; always you must rise
And run like rivers toward the prize.
We live in backwards time today
And count the hours that flew away.
The time to make the greatest stride
Is just the time when strength has died.
The hardest effort must be made
The minute power starts to fade
And when you feel the rush of pride
That rush will carry you astride
And lend you quickness in your pace
To faster run the uphill race
While others work, achieve, and rest
For you, the opposite is best.

Kelly always responded to poetry and music lyrics. I think stories and books have too many characters and plot actions for her to recall. I plan to write my daughter many poems, both good and awful. I realize I should also buy her books filled with great poetry.

Integra - Early '93

I've written that Kelly was attending school for half of the day, seeing the homebound tutor after lunch and going to physical therapy in the late afternoons. Well, she worked relentlessly, seven days a week with no time out for a life. Even in car rides, we would recite multiplication tables for review (forgotten but quickly recalled), Spanish verbs, English poetry. Memorizing data was possible, but took scores of repetitions and time. Time was Kelly's enemy. We needed much longer days.

That spring the Bouldins spent only one day away from academia. We took Kelly to visit an old friend, Holly Bond, in Atlanta, Georgia. Her family had moved there after RJR Nabisco relocated its world headquarters away from "bucolic" Winston-Salem. Kelly seemed to enjoy spending time with her old friend, but after leaving, we started calling out poetry terms in the car. "Onomatopoeia... Shhhhhhhhh!"

When we returned home, Kelly remembered that she had obtained her learner's permit just prior to her injury. I couldn't imagine a child with shaky hands and double vision ever passing the test for a permanent license. I wasn't even sure she should try. Sometimes, my hope monitor was silent.

Then Kelly and I came home from a particularly difficult day at school. She had not received extended time on a vocabulary test and had failed it.

"Whose car is that?" Kelly inquired as I pulled into our garage. On the street beside our house was a bright aquamarine Acura Integra. Both Tyler and Kelly thought Acuras were the ultimate car.

"I have no clue," I answered as her father, Bobby, came out the back door, grinning like a sneaky toddler. He approached Kelly and handed her a set of car keys. She smiled with more animation than I'd seen in months. She zoomed to the car, plopped herself into the driver's seat and turned on the radio, loudly.

I took a deep breath. "Do you really believe she'll ever drive that car?" I asked my husband.

"Sure. And until she can, she can sit out here and play her own music. This will give her a reason to keep fighting. And she will drive the car."

Did you ever notice, in a good marriage, that when one partner is crumbling, the other has a way of picking up the slack and being strong? We'd promised not to let Kelly's TBI wreck our marriage, and for the first time, I knew the promise would be kept.

"Come listen, mom, come see. This is awesome!"

Kelly took ten steps forward that day because she believed she had a future.

5 Uncle Jimmy - '93

"A friend is one before whom I may think aloud."
– Emerson

Sometimes when they are needed the most, the best of friends appear. There may not be many of them, but Dr. James Mattox was definitely one. As my psychiatrist, he listened to me talk endlessly, and he saved me from myself over and over again. Kelly's first Christmas at home had been an abysmal disappointment. Friends did not rush over to visit; she was bored, often in pain, confused, and in my opinion, deeply depressed. Her right hand shook like an eggbeater, and she had gained about twenty pounds from eating "easy to swallow" foods, which were high in carbohydrates. The weather seemed angry, as it was cold and gray outside. This reflected my personal outlook on life. At a check-up for Kelly, Dr. McWhorter looked at me and said, "You need Uncle Jimmy."

Dr. McWhorter had been Dr. James Mattox's (Jimmy's) roommate in medical school. Now, depression is not a subject I would ever approach lightly. My elder brother Tom, a successful orthodontist, had died by his own hand a few years previously. Yet I hesitated to take Kelly to see a psychiatrist. She already felt abnormal and was struggling to regain an identity as a regular, healthy teenager. Anyway, I made an appointment and went alone for my first psychiatric evaluation.

Dr. James Mattox reminded me of Santa Claus. He fixed me sugared coffee and we both lit a cigarette. I said, "I have two questions."

"Shoot," he said.

"Is it all right for me to be here just to tell you about my daughter Kelly? This way you'll be prepared when she realizes she needs help."

"Do you have other children?" he responded. I told him yes and he continued. "All of your family may need help because a severe traumatic brain injury in one family member affects everyone."

"Tyler will be fine," I answered quickly, not wanting the conversation to deviate from Kelly. "She's in college and I doubt Bobby, my husband, would be willing to visit a psychiatrist."

"What's your other question?" he said, obviously worried about Tyler.

"My family has a history of depression and my brother committed suicide. Does this mean that I need to be evaluated myself?"

"Yes."

And so we began. In that first hour, I learned much about myself as well as TBI and its aftermath. Jimmy asked me to write down three times when I had been truly happy. I wrote: a family vacation in the Bahamas, my children winning swim relays years ago on my July birthday, and just walking on the beaches of North and South Carolina.

"Is this cold, dark weather getting you down, and are you sleeping?" he asked.

"Yes. No."

"You have SAD, or Seasonal Affective Disorder," said Jimmy. "It can run in families, like depression can."

Anyway, cups of coffee later, I walked out feeling oddly calm. I now had my back door—someone Kelly could run to if I was impaired, unavailable or ill-equipped. I hoped she would use this back door someday. I began taking the anti-depressant Paxil the next day, and it helped. Dr. Mattox taught me the reason to seek therapy Post Trauma. "You need to talk about your fears and pain," he said, "but the person you talk to needs to be able to sleep at night. I can, but your family members won't be able to." I'm so glad Uncle Jimmy came into our lives. Hopefully Kelly will want to meet him someday.

Completing The Freshman Year: '92 - '93

With the homebound help of Ms. Gibson, Kelly finally completed 2nd semester freshman Spanish, science, history, and English. With the tutorial help of Nancy Bearden, she completed two semesters of Spanish. With my help and her own determination, she completed her first semester courses.

P. E. was another matter. After battles with the administration of the high school, Kelly was finally allowed to use rehabilitation time spent at The Martinat Center (outpatient rehabilitation center) and the YMCA as her P.E. requirement for those two terms. There were always so many battles for such small but vital things, yet Kelly proudly set the precedent in Forsyth County for using physical therapy (PT) hours as credit in physical education.

I told the school, "If Charlotte-Mecklenburg County allows physical therapy to count as P.E., then Forsyth County should, too." Guidance agreed, and these credit hours allowed Kelly to be a sophomore in 1993-94. The truth was, I didn't know what Charlotte-Mecklenburg did, but the precedent was still set. One small step for students with TBI.

Against all odds, Kelly didn't fall behind her class despite her severe closed-head injury!

The Sky is Falling

In June of '93, Bobby and I took a group of girls to Ocean Isle Beach, figuring if we paid for it, some of Kelly's newer high school friends would agree to come. Sometimes I could almost feel sorry for the 14 to 15-year-old girls who just didn't know how to deal with Kelly's problems; but most of the time, I resented their disappearance from her life the past spring. They had wanted her to return from rehab miraculously healed. These girls were not prepared for, old enough, or patient enough for a long, long convalescence.

At the beach I saw them try to transform Kelly into her old self, and in a way, this was positive. They wrapped Kelly's shaking right arm in a bandage, and told the boys they met that she had a soccer injury.

"It worked!" Carla yelled. The group had been to an arcade down the street to flirt with boys. Kelly had played, and was happy that no one knew of her TBI. Pool and golf were her two left-handed sports. This trip was turning out to be socially positive, until the phone rang and I got what I had wished for.

The first night at the beach I had walked outside to the ocean, and just listened to the waves crashing against the shore. I remembered my English class from high school and a fragment of a Langston Hughes poem called "The Island":

Wave if sorrow
Do not drown me now,
I see the island
Still ahead somehow...

I felt lonely. I wished that one other mother could be my true peer and know the pain of losing a child. The next morning I got my wish—my horrible, life-altering wish. The phone rang, and my friend Diane gave the news:

"One of the girls' friends died last night. It was Britt. He had a heart attack in the car, and crashed into a tree. Bring the girls home!"

Kelly had lost the one friend who knew what high school was like if you had a disability, and you couldn't party and drink. On the long ride home with a car full of sobbing teenagers, I had my first full-fledged panic attack and had to pull off the road to breathe and stop crying.

Britt Armfield had been born with a congenital heart defect, and had undergone open-heart surgery to repair any defects; however, the medication he was taking failed to prevent the ventricular tachycardia he was experiencing. Tragically, at age sixteen he suffered a fatal heart attack at the wheel of a car. He was not supposed to leave us, and his precious mother Prissy was not supposed to share my pain. Kelly was dumbstruck by Britt's death.

"I miss Britt. I miss sitting with him in the hospital. I miss knowing that he knows what being different is like. I should be dead instead of Britt. God took the wrong person!"

Kelly would turn to her computer, and slowly type out her pain.

A Lesson From Britt - Summer '93

Kelly was devastated by the loss of Britt, who understood her more than any other peer. She wanted to show his parents, Ed and Prissy, the letter Britt sent to the hospital when she was in coma. We all soon learned that Ed Armfield was dying of cancer, and he seemed to enjoy Kelly's frequent visits—he would soon be with his son, and Kelly loved him, too.

One day we learned Ed was on his way into a surgery; Kelly grabbed a framed picture of herself and made me drive her to the hospital. We found the Armfields as Ed was being rolled into surgery. She put her picture on his chest and said, "You won't die today."

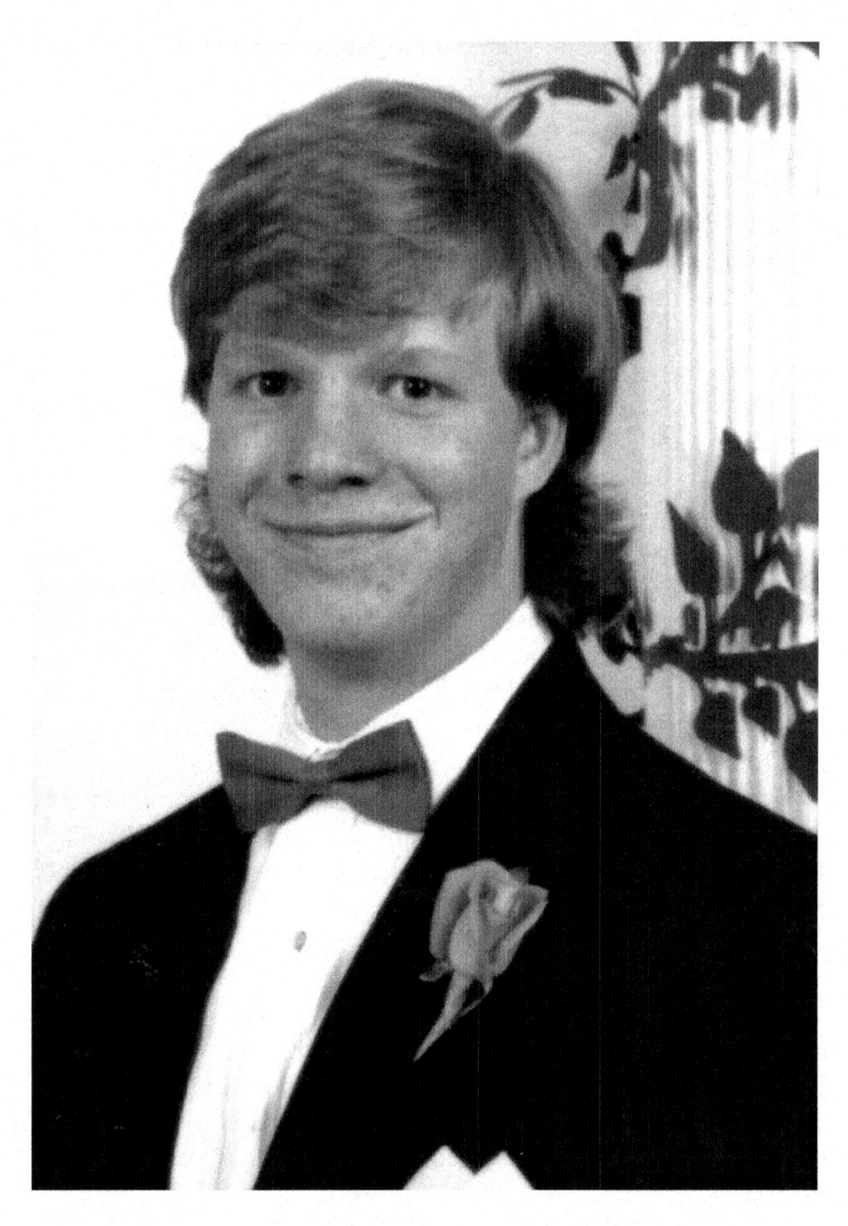

Britt Armfield, August 4th, 1976 – June 12th, 1993

"You're my angel," he said. And Ed Armfield did survive that surgery, but died soon after. Such visits helped Kelly learn that she could still make a tiny difference in the lives of others. She could still be useful, even if she couldn't be exactly like other teenagers. Prissy Armfield, who lost both a son and a husband in one year, allowed Kelly to spend many hours with her. Bless her for letting Kelly know she still had strength.

With Prissy's help, the summer of '93 changed Kelly's inward focus to an outer one. Consequently, the summer became a time of giving attention to other sick children and their caretakers. For instance, one of Kelly's friends had a severe case of mononucleosis (a.k.a mono). Kelly (with help) delivered balloons and videos for her friend to watch while convalescing. My daughter spent several hours commiserating with the boy and left feeling a genuine sense of accomplishment. Kelly so desperately needed to be needed by her friends again. Our home was now too filled with silence. The phone had long since stopped its constant ringing.

Even going back to visit Kelly's nurses and other sick children at Brenner's was a way to pass the time and also give Kelly real purpose. One afternoon we knocked on the *staff only* door of the 5th floor ICU where Kelly spent eleven days. No one came so we just walked in. Immediately we saw a wonderful ICU nurse named Doris, who had cared for my child. And she remembered.

"Kelly!" she exclaimed, looking into her eyes. "Your lights are on! We don't often see that!" Doris meant, of course, that the blank stare of new patients with TBI is common, and some never recover their connection to reality. "It's so good to see the light in your eyes," Doris went on. "Most people never come back to visit us in the ICU... thank you so much for coming... you have made my day!"

Another special visit I remember: Once we paid a call on a friend of my husband, Pebble Wall (his real name). Pebble had suffered an open-head TBI in an automobile accident near Chapel Hill. Post-surgery, he was now convalescing at home. Pebble loved golf, and he asked Kelly, "If I try to hit a golf ball now, do you think I can do it? Or will I hit the dirt?"

She answered calmly and candidly, "You'll hit the dirt!" They both laughed and hugged each other. Pebble was Kelly's first TBI peer.

A little advice? If you happen to be the parent of an adolescent child with TBI, do not waste time regretting the wild and crazy parties your child won't be able to attend on the weekends. Kelly developed a personal motto: On any day that you can't be happy, make at least one other person happy. Although most of her time was spent in therapy sessions or studying something forgotten, Kelly managed to fill her free hours by focusing more on those in need. Perhaps we'll always hate holidays and weekends, as we remember our constant battle to stave off boredom and loneliness during the lulls in school; but Kelly will always know how important it is to give her love and time to others.

Jurassic Park - Summer '93

Because of Kelly's vision problems, I spent hours every day reading to her, both her homework and pleasure reading. Unfortunately, she couldn't remember the beginning of a story by the time we reached the ending, so fiction made little sense. Once or twice we'd attempted to watch a movie together, but she grew bored, unable to focus on the plots and characters for long. Then in June of 1993, the movie *Jurassic Park* became popular with her friends, and she asked to go. I took her alone because Kelly's driving peers were often afraid to ride with her along. This movie became meaningful to me, to us, because for the first time, Kelly followed every twist of the plot for two whole hours. However, the vocabulary sometimes escaped her. As the children in the film worried about the approach of escaped dinosaurs, Kelly asked in an extremely loud voice: "What the hell is a T-Rex?" Some people laughed out loud, but a high school friend named Stuart Welch came to sit next to Kelly. He explained terminology and seemed to enjoy helping her comprehend. Stuart didn't mind Kelly's loudness or her lack of knowledge. He simply helped out, and made a world of difference to her on both social and cognitive levels.

6 Sophomore Year: '93-'94

The academic year of 1993-1994 was Kelly's first full-time school year post-trauma, and we learned she couldn't have corrective eye surgery for two more years. Dr. Weaver, her eye surgeon, wanted to see if her double vision would self-correct. Thus Kelly, with her numerous problems, tackled public high school full-time with a normal load of classes. At times, it seemed like it tackled her. Mr. Mock, guidance counselor, helped us choose classes we thought she could handle.

Kelly, with assistance from Mr. Mock and me, chose to enroll in an Honors level English class, as did many of her friends. The English teacher was my friend, and agreed to monitor Kelly's progress both socially and educationally in this challenging program.

Kelly needed many assignments read to her, and would eventually turn in three types of writing. "D" indicated "dictated," and on a dictated paper, I typed exactly what she told me to type. Then there were her worst papers, which were barely legible, handwritten and shaky. Finally, there were those she typed alone on the word processor. The dictated efforts were naturally the best, but I love each of her writings and treasure them still.

One day at the high school, I heard a teacher say, "Frankenstein is coming." I realized quickly she was talking about me. I was, in her eyes, a Dr. Frankenstein who was trying to create a life that couldn't exist in reality. Was I pushing Kelly too hard, too fast, in school? I called Dr. McWhorter and asked him if I'd made the wrong decision.

"Should I be preparing Kelly for a normal life? Or should I take her out of a difficult school situation and prepare her for the life of someone permanently impaired?"

He said, "You have no choice to make. I have never met a person who could do anything they didn't believe they could do." So I kept

Kelly in high school in honors classes. I would be Frankenstein and embrace the title.

Why did I continue to keep Kelly in an advanced academic program? Because her friends were there, and she needed to regain her memories. Because she gave me "little gifts" every day, which indicated advanced thinking. For instance, I read her Shakespeare's comedy, *The Tempest*, because her eyes couldn't focus on the small textbook print. I stopped often, asking her questions about her understanding of Prospero's island antics.

At the end, she said: "This is not a comedy. It's a tragedy. The king gave up his magic for a silly teenage girl."

I had never told her that *The Tempest* was Shakespeare's farewell to the theatre, his last play. Indeed, the story had tragic elements. The island magic was ending. Kelly's remarks like this one kept me pushing her into harder classes, when basic classes might have been far simpler and less stressful. But I wanted my whole child back, and I believe she wanted the same.

At about this time Kelly chose to switch from being right-handed to being permanently left-handed. For months, she had written by grasping her right wrist to hold the right hand steady, and only then was she able to write to some degree. Students had begun to make lewd jokes about Kelly's jerky hand motions, so one day she came home and said, "I don't care what Dr. Kelly says. I won't use my right hand anymore. It's staying in my pocket!" And so she began a long process of change. Her "78s" became "87s" for a time, but she persevered. At home she continued to practice with the right hand, but for school, she never used it again.

Catch 22: Doctors Vs. Rules - '93-'94

Both of Kelly's primary doctors had recommended that Kelly do school assignments on a laptop computer. Sadly, they didn't communicate much with her high school. First, they asked for her to take a course in keyboarding. Kelly had taken one such class in junior high, but taking another would hopefully stimulate both her tactile and kinesthetic memories. The keyboarding teacher refused to put Kelly in her class, stating, "She won't be able to keep up!"

The same doctors who wanted Kelly to take a keyboarding class strongly advised her to take an art class as therapy for a bilateral hand impairment. After the initial class this teacher responded, "She can't keep up." She went so far as to threaten Kelly with a "guaranteed F" if we dared keep Kelly in her class. I was called to a conference with this woman in September, and shown Kelly's blossoming portfolio. There emerged one perfect, beautiful ivy leaf, with veins and appropriate shading! I cried, because I didn't know she could do it. My daughter could still draw, even with her left hand. Yet the art teacher mocked her efforts.

"There should have been nine to twelve leaves in this picture!" she said coldly. "Kelly hasn't done enough work to even receive a grade." My response was a whisper, "I hope you die."

So I took Kelly out of art class, from a subject that could have motivated her and saved the family a fortune in occupational therapy sessions. I found myself thinking, "OK, the art major is out." Well, hadn't the principal told us that once we returned from Myers Lake Rehab, Kelly could have anything she needed from her high school? We quickly learned that promises were just words and could be forgotten as quickly as they left one's mouth. Administrators clearly had to cope with a staff unfamiliar with TBI. Part of me sympathized. Most of me wished I'd gotten all promises in writing.

However, after much thinking and advice from Mr. Mock, chorus turned out to be the best alternative to art, although Kelly could barely talk, much less sing. She was still having trouble with her vocal chords. Words and syllables were coming slowly, with a flat monotone sound. She was struggling to vary the pitch of her words, even to the point of practicing speech in front of a mirror.

At any rate, the chorus teacher, benevolent Terry Hicks, provided a sanctuary for Kelly in his chorus room. He helped her to sing note by note, and made sure she could hide in his room during stressful moments in the school day. Mr. Hicks wins my medal for most compassionate teacher at R.J. Reynolds High School. He even assigned compassionate students like Ashley Knight to gently push Kelly onto stage during choral performances, because she would forget her cues.

The academic pace for Kelly (and me) was grueling. We tried sending Kelly to a math tutor, but while she would understand concepts, she'd forget them in two hours. So I started seeing the tutor as well. I would then come home and stay up all night putting problems on poster paper, to make them large enough for Kelly's eyes to see. That system worked, for her math skills seemed less harmed. She was making A's in math at least.

Other subjects were much harder, as my child was attempting to memorize Greek and Roman history. Kelly was also relearning world geography so that countries of similar size and shape weren't confusing. Amnesia is strange. One can remember the more difficult concepts like theorems and still wonder, "Who the hell are Matthew, Mark, Luke, and John?" or "What the heck is a geranium?" which Kelly asked me one afternoon. It was always so hard to know what Kelly didn't know. But she, at least, asked the questions.

Kelly did, however, have one true friend who always helped her. Nicole never seemed to mind how embarrassing or tactless my child was, and for that loyalty, I am forever grateful. Kelly even wrote a poem about Nicole's friendship at Christmas in 1993:

Someone

Someone who is happy and joyful, yet sincere
Who fills your life with beauty and cheer
Someone who grieves and comforts, yet smiles
Who wants to spend time with you for awhile
Someone who is there if you need a friend
Who will support and defend you, again and again
Someone who helps you and keeps their love sound
Who is loyal and caring, and will always be around
Someone whose strength will help you stand
Who will not hesitate to lend you a hand
Someone whose love will always stay true
Someone special, someone like you.

Nicole Price and Suzanne Davis remained constant friends while others vanished, but even they were confused by the mood swings of a convalescent with TBI. After writing "Someone" for Nicole, she handed me this lovely poem, "Again," written with her trembling right hand.

Mother [illegible]
I look around and I see,
inumerable things I want to
experience,
countless things I would like
to be.
People walk through life with
their eyes closed. [illegible]
Never looking around,
At what might be discovered.
Without you I would be blind,
Never knowing what to see,
You've kept me ALIVE!
And helped me find me,
AGAIN.

Again (handwritten draft)

Cheerleading *Again:* Sophomore Year

Unfortunately, the issue of a student with TBI cheering came up again early sophomore year. This year a "basketball-only" squad was being selected. Relentless, Kelly was practicing jumps and cheers whenever she had a spare minute. She even allowed me to videotape her jumps, her falling—a thing she loathed last year—to see how she could improve. The tapes always reminded her of her deficits. I was surprised at her willingness to study her own gait, her slower movements, her progress.

This year I discussed the issue of cheering with high school administration. I soon received a letter advising that Kelly needed "further tests" before try-outs.

The following letter responds to the school system's request to have Kelly do well on an IQ test before becoming a basketball cheerleader. If that sounds a bit odd to the reader, that's because it was. The request was a blatant dodge by those who feared liability from a child recovering from brain injuries. That's just my informed opinion.

12/29/1993

> To the Winston-Salem/Forsyth County Schools:
>
> Thank you for taking the time to talk to Bob and me about our daughter's problems following a traumatic brain injury. In a letter to (certain school employees, unnamed) on 11/15/92, we requested immediate help in restoring Kelly to her prior physical activity of J.V. cheerleading, in order to stimulate her brain and motor skills, and thus her overall recovery. A member (via a conversation 12/28/1992) of the neuropsychological team of Bowman Gray Hospital confirmed our opinion that such physical stimulation could enhance and stimulate Kelly's mind in other areas.
>
> It would seem that there is indecision on how to handle one of North Carolina's first students classified TBI. We told Ms. S. that, in order to help Kelly, Thanksgiving would be a deadline for a decision to reinstate her to her squad. Now we have been offered a date of January 26th for a neurological (not a physical) examination to ascertain her strength and coordination. At the taxpayer's expense, this examination would be yet another IQ test, and hardly a judge of her ability to cheer for her team. Regardless, the basketball season would be nearly

> over by the time she completed this test; thus we must accept your proposal as a denial to reinstate her.
>
> We would have been glad to comply with the recommended testing for Kelly had the test been offered in time for her to have trained with her squad. As it is, we will not use the school system's money to undergo post facto tests.
>
> Without doubt this situation will arise again. I can only wish that soon you can all agree to make speedy and timely decisions that can benefit children with traumatic brain injuries; especially those, like Kelly, who have received medical clearance from their physicians to participate in certain activities. Our family hopes that, in the future, you will try to ensure that children with TBI are allowed to become re-immersed in their old and familiar activities. As an LD teacher and the mother of a child who suffered TBI, I can assure you that this is the way to ensure the most complete recovery.
>
> Sincerely yours,
> Carolyn and Robert Bouldin

I asked an official for the school system if he truly wanted me to use taxpayer dollars, about $3,000, for tests in January 1993 that might indicate a high enough IQ for a cheerleader (I was laughing at the time). He said, "Yes." He spoke to me in a hallway where no one else could hear. My bluff had been called, and I realized I needed to keep learning the political system of the public schools better in order to help Kelly in the future.

After a second failure, in spring '94, Kelly tried out one last time for cheerleading, and I was totally exhausted. She'd kept us up most of the night reviewing moves, practicing jumps, falling, repeating moves, until she had actually memorized the short routine. At school I was not allowed to enter the gym to watch the actual try-outs, but she soon ran out of the building and leapt into the car with my sister and me. I drove away, looking at her tragic face in the rearview mirror.

About a block from the high school, she rolled down the car window and threw her favorite ring out into a yard. She then took off her cheer jacket from last year and threw that away also. I pulled the car over. My sister Clara walked back into the yard and found the silver horse-shaped ring that had been Kelly's most prized possession. She left the jacket. Kelly came home, went into her room, and smashed every mirror in sight, and I let her. Later she repeated her motto, "ten steps forward, two steps backwards." She couldn't cry, but her entire body shook with anger and pain.

I will never forget how hard she worked on cheers in that spring, learning them all, forgetting so much faster, learning again. I remember the flat angry tone of her voice, "What exactly do I have to do to be on the squad again? Doesn't anyone understand how much I need this?"

Why were we surprised she wasn't chosen, ever?

My rational mind now tells me Kelly was lucky to return to a public high school so soon after her TBI. I'm sure the staff worried about knowing what to do with her. Yet, somehow I feel that they failed Kelly by keeping her away from familiar activities.

I am beyond angry and I don't think anyone cares. Like Kelly, I have no peers.

Escaping and Growing

By the summer of 1994, Kelly was closing in on the two-year mark post-TBI. Doctors, family, and Kelly herself decided she needed a change of scenery in a controlled environment. She applied (with my help) to be a counselor-in-training (CIT) at Camp Thunderbird near Charlotte, NC. We had all decided not to tell them of Kelly's condition. Therefore, with no medical red tape, she was accepted and spent one month as a CIT in a place full of kids. There were no cars and no alcohol or drugs to my knowledge.

The day we arrived, Kelly and I simply told the camp nurse about her TBI history. I assured her that Kelly could be a good counselor's helper in putting eight-year-olds to bed each night. Kelly was also assigned to assist the cheerleading coach during the day, and the little children loved her. At Thunderbird Kelly still felt different from the other CITs, but she made many new friends, and most importantly, she realized that there was a world outside of Winston-Salem. As a CIT, your parents had to pay the same tuition as a regular camper (the age to be a CIT is sixteen). Thus our little subterfuge was cheating no one. The camp evidently was pleased with Kelly, for no one ever said a negative world about my neglecting to mention her handicaps, although her hands were still shaking.

The day Kelly returned home, I invited a group of her friends over, and when I speak of Kelly's friends, I'm not referring to the seemingly fair-weather ones she had before her accident. The friends I'm speaking of were either the childhood friends she had grown up with, or newly acquired friends. When the large group arrived, we put a "Welcome

Home" banner over her bed. The one month Kelly had spent away was a turning point in her confidence level and in her recovery as a whole. Her friends seemed a bit dismayed that she could accomplish such a long summer job. I was thrilled, as I had daily expected a "come and get me" call. But she survived it, even though the experience was very difficult for her. I found a poem which reflected the fear she must have felt away from home:

Thunderbird

I am at a place without any friends.
I am happy, but when will this end?
My friends don't write.
I wonder where they are.
I miss my parents, my friends, and my car.
Bennett's a guy that I'm interested in.
But I can't tell what's happening.
Are we just friends?
Sometimes I worry, as I ponder and stare.
Does he like me, or do I care?
It's hard not to worry when you miss things so much.
Yet camp is awesome, or is thought of as such.
I want to go home, yet I want to stay.
I'm indecisive, confused, or just "messed up" that way.
I will decide, if I dare.
No.
I remain apathetic, which means I don't care.

Family Crisis - '94

In Homer's *Iliad*, Zeus makes a display of his famous urns. The *Two Urns of Zeus* are filled with blessings for mankind, and alternately, with hardships and demonic evils. The king of the gods, according to Homer, enjoyed pouring upon humans from whichever urn struck his fancy. *"Good...bad....hmm, a little more bad today."* Truly this view of divinity makes some sense to me, more so at times than the Christian view of a merciful god who rewards hard work and virtue. At any rate, I came home from the grocery store, facing about eight hours of Kelly homework and another doctor's appointment. The answering machine was blinking. I punched the button. "Bob, so sorry to hear you won't be with the company any longer. Rotten break, Call me." No. Could my husband, head of a company, have lost his job?

Why, sure. I don't live on the right side of the looking glass anymore. Why not?

It turned out that the president of Bob's company granted him several weeks of paid time off to help out with Kelly's rehab. My husband was told to release several customers whose business ties weren't that important. Bob did as he was told, and the Chairman of the Board of his company reversed the decision of the company president. Profits being more important than people, Bob Bouldin was released. Zeus dumped more evil upon us, and the Bouldins were now unemployed. Kelly's insurance couldn't be settled until she was 18, and the bills kept rolling in. I couldn't express how I felt, but anger and hate are words that pale in comparison to my actual murderous state of mind.

Amazing Men - '94

Kelly, you may never publish an account of your early post-TBI days. You may remember your parents as slave drivers who tortured you into studying and exercising beyond human limits. I don't even expect you to forgive us completely for the torments we forced you to endure. If your love is the price to pay for your recovery, I can handle it.

However, I do want you to someday look back and realize that your father is the most amazing man. For many months, Bob got up at his regular time, dressed for work, and went to the public library to read and research employment opportunities. You thought he was going to work as usual. He didn't want to add anxiety to your life, and never told you of his job loss until he was employed elsewhere. Watching him leave each day, in complete suit and tie, made me remember why I married Bobby in the first place. He is the best of fathers, putting your well-being before his own. If you climb out of this well you are drowning in, your father will be the one pulling on the rope!

Learning to Drive - '94

Bobby told me later he would never have tried so hard to teach Kelly to drive if he had known how badly her vision was impaired. She was good at hiding her problems. Like any sixteen-year-old, she wanted to drive a car. Each afternoon, at about five o'clock, Bobby would let Kelly drive her new Acura around one or two blocks near our home. The car would weave badly, as Kelly steered with shaking hands. She also had to close one eye to allow for single vision. My daughter, as stubborn as ever, refused to wear her eye patch because it made her look different. On the road she either drove too close to the center line, or too close to parked cars nearby. When parking, she smashed a lot of hubcaps. Bobby had given up drinking when doctors told us that even small amounts of alcohol could kill Kelly, but he began to take swigs of bourbon before each driving lesson.

Eventually this gruesome twosome attempted to pass the licensure test. Doctors warned us not to tell the Division of Motor Vehicles about her TBI, because the restrictions involved could follow her long after further recovery.

"Should I drive with my left hand because it shakes less?" Kelly asked.

"Let's try it," her dad said. She failed that first test because she didn't use both hands on the wheel. The next week she and her father went to a different branch of the DMV. Kelly used both hands, but told the official, "I had a soccer injury to my right hand, and it's shaking." She came home triumphant. "I passed!" Of course we couldn't let her drive anywhere alone. Even with us in the car, she was a threat to humanity. But merely gaining the license was another "ten steps forward" for Kelly. Now we just had to sit back and wait to see what the two steps back would entail.

My husband became a good player in the teenager game. He often planned business trips where Kelly and a friend could go along. This would give Kelly a feeling of camaraderie without letting her know the true intent. As time passed, my child was healing.

Reflections

Young Life of America was the best organization to help Kelly during her high school years. Young Life is a non-denominational Christian ministry committed to making a difference in kids' lives through friendships with caring adults. She went on several trips to Windy Gap, a camp in the mountains of North Carolina. She even traveled to Young Life's Pioneer Ranch in Colorado, with leaders watching closely over her. In Colorado, she went rafting down a river, with double vision, a mere nine months after her accident. There had been a Young Life leader on each side of her, so she had been fairly safe. She climbed to the top of a mountain on the same trip, shaming many far stronger teens into completing the climb. Again she was kept safe by leaders supporting her every step.

I remember my daughter telling me that her single vision returned from certain angles on the top of that mountain in Colorado. She said to me: "Britt was there climbing the mountain. I wanted to stop. I was tired, but he told me to keep going. I got to the top, looked up at the sky, and I could see only *one sun*." This and her other trips away from home terrified me, but they gave Kelly a much-needed sense of confidence in herself.

By the end of the third year post-TBI, Kelly was performing work crew jobs at the Young Life camp in Windy Gap, NC.

By mid-high school, Kelly actually became very adept at forming new friendships during lunches, mostly with new students unfamiliar with Winston-Salem. Kelly hated seeing kids left out. She befriended Caroline Manner, and others new to town. Caring for others had always been a Kelly trait, and I saw this reasserting itself. She began to ask new friends home, or to attend ball games. However, she was also learning of all the things she couldn't do anymore. What she sorely needed was to discover a handful of activities at which she could excel. The only problem was that there wasn't anything. Kelly couldn't find out who she was from doctors, as they offered differing opinions.

I functioned as her scribe while she dictated lessons. I saw her mind growing and healing. I couldn't give her 20-20 vision to read with, or steady hands to paint with. I just tried to be patient with my little girl who once said at age two, "I hate patience!"

I'd been an LD (Learning Disabilities) language therapist for many years, and was used to seeking different pathways or new, creative methods for reaching a student who seemed unable to learn a concept by standard methods. I still believe that with persistent effort, a brain-injured person can be taught something when standard procedure fails.

For instance, in teaching Kelly geometry, I relied on her kinesthetic sense (motion). I would draw the triangle and angles with the arc of her arms. I would explain theorems using her arms as line segments. The motion triggered informed responses when verbal instruction failed. I.e., her body's movements helped her establish a new pathway for information. Kelly made an A in geometry after beginning the semester with an F. I had made a D- in this subject myself in high school. But late nights and will power forced me to finally learn this subject.

The best advice when a topic seems unlearnable: find a new way to present it, a way that stimulates many senses. Kelly found out for herself, and then told me that she learned best after physical stimulation. She learned this playing pool. After a few shots, she could memorize data that earlier eluded her. I was constantly questioning my child's doctors to verify the validity of physical stimulation affecting recall. One confirmed our hypothesis that by stimulating her body, Kelly was probably also stimulating her mind and ability to memorize. The downside to this was huge fatigue levels following the exercise-then-learning routine, but the results were worth it.

My daughter was and is a fighter. If she hadn't helped me to help her, and been willing to accept my assistance, her recovery would have been slowed. Thank you, brave daughter, for having patience with me and working with me during your teenage years when time spent with one's parents is not very desirable!

"Geometry is what makes me know I'm not stupid," she once told me.

There was comfort in the routine of figuring things out logically, things not memorized but analyzed. There were teachers who tapped into the old and new Kelly, like Mr. Warren (math) and Mr. Walls (history). They would trigger back the old memories, always teaching, not always grading, measuring, comparing. They allowed Kelly to take tests until she could pass them. She was able to number geometric theorems instead of writing out their definitions, and solve proofs in a numeric shorthand. I thank them.

Kelly spent every minute proving something. "I can hop now. I can drive now. I can write left-handed now. I can cheer now, but I don't know who I am or who my friends are. Look at me, my hair has grown back from where it was shaved in the hospital. No, I don't want to date. Too much stress involved. Too much stress to trust people."

Doctors guessed after many months that Kelly might be able to "go to college someday." We'll save for her continuing psychiatric needs. Sadly, victims of TBI can become suicidal, and I knew Kelly had fallen too far to be immune from depression.

Dr. Kelly once told me, "It's almost tragic that she remembers her excellence." But I was beginning to discover something about amnesia: a Type A personality can survive a traumatic brain injury, or perhaps a Type B is forced to become Type A... this new Kelly was simply not giving up!

Part Two: Kelly Speaks

Part Two: Kelly Speaks is written in Kelly's voice and portrays her memories of life, both in and out of Academia, with a traumatic brain injury (TBI). Any statistical errors regarding the prevalence of TBI are unintentional as the numbers are constantly rising.

7 Going Back to School

"Nothing ever comes to one, that is worth having, except as a result of hard work."

—Booker T. Washington

My parents often told me of my accomplishments in high school which impressed and, at times, amazed them. Going to Pioneer Ranch in Colorado and to Windy Gap alone, or with no one directly supervising me, were two examples that especially pleased them. My parents were aware of people laughing at me behind my back, and were thrilled that I still had the courage to continue on with my life, seemingly unfazed. At the time, I knew some of the things people were saying and doing. My slow speech or aphasia was easy to mimic. My gait was clearly amusing to copy. But not having the power to change people's perceptions, I had no other choice but to continue on, always moving forward. As my swollen brain healed, my ability to remember bits and pieces came slowly back. Without the memories of close friends and family, I wouldn't comprehend the first few years following my confrontation with a telephone pole; but through reading their notes and hearing their stories, some memories have actually returned.

I do remember what going back to school was like in 1992-1993, yet I cannot explain it as well as I would like to. My feelings are vague, but real. I thought high school would make me happy, and my life would return to normalcy. Yet my body betrayed my desires.

What did I want, need, when I returned home post-TBI? I try to remember my altered life at age 15...

I wanted what all teenagers want from their parents—privacy! When I look back at 1992, I remember anger, even rage, at a mother who slept in my room. Yes, I was relearning how to walk. But "I don't care if I fall! I can always crawl!" I screamed at her most nights. She remained at my side anyway, making sure I didn't stumble in the night, always grasping some part of my body that yearned for separation.

And when I think harder, I remember blood, obscuring other sensations that once brought happiness.

The first Christmas back home in late '92, all I wanted was solitude. The house was decorated with mistletoe and wreaths, coupled with the smells of pine from the Christmas tree, and hot gingerbread emanating from the kitchen. Amongst feelings of warmth and family, which enveloped me constantly, I also felt like the center of everyone's attention.

I mostly wanted to be left alone, and I certainly didn't require an audience to watch me cleanse myself. My mother shaved my legs for me, and I hated her for it. Placing a beach towel on the floor, she rubbed lotion onto my legs and carefully shaved them. My hands shook terribly then, like a man drilling through concrete. But I so desired to shave my own legs... just once. Finally my mother ran me a deep bath and promised to leave me alone to soak and relax for thirty minutes. Wow, what a wonderful gift, an early Christmas present... I loved her for understanding my need for freedom. I took my portable CD player in the bathroom, and allowed mother to hold me as I sank down deep into water filled with purple and pink bubbles, smelling of musty lilac. Then she was really, truly gone, and I was finally, thankfully alone.

Then I saw it. The razor on the ledge. And I knew I could do it myself. I didn't like rough, hairy legs, and didn't care if I cut myself shaving. Inch by inch, I shaved my legs, steadying my right hand while holding that wrist with the left hand.

And I bled. But it didn't hurt at all, so I kept going and bled a little more. If I cut a vein or artery, who would care? I didn't.

Then I looked down into the water instead of upwards at the leg on the bathtub ledge – a crimson pool. For an instant, I couldn't breathe. I lay in a shallow tub of bloody water. I had been so incredibly happy before.... Soon my mother came back, clasped the door... and screamed.

I don't remember Christmas day, but I do have a three-inch scar over my shinbone on my left leg to remind me of the incident. Following that 30 minutes of freedom, I begrudgingly agreed to mom's heavy and constant surveillance.

Another memory I banished to the deepest, most remote part of my brain is that of bruises. I can remember staring in a full-length mirror on the back of my bedroom door, and counting the number of bruises and scratches covering my naked body. The countless cheerleading jumps attempted in front of my parents' house always resulted in bruising and sometimes bloody finishes. I tripped and fell frequently in the time following my TBI and before undergoing eye surgery. Afraid of heights, I still have the occasional nightmare involving the third story of Reynolds High School, where I trip at the top of the stairs and reach out for a missing banister.

But falling down in stairwells was solely my fault. Desperate for independence and receiving little at home, I rushed out of classes and refused help from anyone who offered. I can recall friends who said, "I'll be glad to carry your books, Kelly. Want to hold my hand?"

"I'm fine... I don't need your help!" I replied regularly. I didn't want anyone to know I was unsure of my next destination. Without consulting the class schedule pasted into my day planner, I had no idea, from hour to hour, where I should be going next. And if I left my book bag and day planner in the last classroom, which I often did, only then would I finally accept a bystander's assistance. So I fell a lot, probably three times a day. My bruises multiplied. There was enough of the stubborn "old Kelly" in me then, to believe I would regain all of my lost abilities quickly, with little time spent in physical or occupational therapy.

I was also foolishly certain of getting on the cheer squad the following year. Of course, I was already doomed by the liability issues involved in school sports. The coaches didn't want to take responsibility for a stumbling, half-blind wreck victim. Today I try not to blame them, but I did in the spring of '93 when I went to school part-time. I still blamed the cheer coaches in my sophomore year. While I know now that TBI was a mystery to staff, I remained angry for months. My bruises were prevalent, both inside and out. At times, the anger exploded, and I would smash furniture and play music loudly to calm myself.

I worried about health problems which kept interrupting my transition back to school. When I brushed my teeth, a simple enough task for most people, I had to push hard with the brush against the gums to keep the brush inside my mouth. Later I learned that Dilantin, an anti-seizure medication I took in 1992, contributed to the recession of my gums, as if someone knew all I needed was just one more thing to deal with. So I had surgery on my gums. I had skin grafted from healthier sections to cover the receded portions. Doctors informed me then that the skin which was grafted might or might not hold, or could hold for several years before receding again.

Like the scar hidden on my scalp from pressure monitor insertion, I have hidden wounds in my mouth. My scars are all concealed, yet I gladly take these permanent badges of honor with me to remind me of where I've been—and where I'm going. Scars give a person personality.

I was frequently scarred at school as well, and those internal wounds are the most painful. Yes, I remember the bad more than the good. The brain does that.

I know that friends would either avoid or, at times, make fun of me. I had to walk looking downward to see where I was going. If I looked up or straight ahead, there were two of everything and I couldn't figure out which vision was real. After a time, I learned to just aim in the middle and that usually worked. Perhaps I was worth laughing at. I began to develop a slumping stature due to the way I was forced to walk, and because of this, people would either mock me or try to emulate my poor posture. I can remember the giggling behind my back. I'd like to forget comments like, "Wow, Kelly's looking rough!"

Following my return to high school, I had to attend numerous meetings concerning my Individualized Education Program, or IEP, where officials discussed me like an object, talking about me as if I were not in the room. I learned that even with an IEP, my teachers at times wouldn't follow or abide by it. "No" was a word I heard often.

I chose to hide from friends who were asked to walk beside of me from class to class. Peer babysitters made me feel very different from my classmates. My walkers were there to keep me from falling and to make sure I made it to class on time. I remember thinking horses and dogs used walkers, and theirs was a service I definitely didn't want or require.

I got lost and fell down steps several times a week. I turned my nose up at the administration's suggestions of help, I guess, but I'd been an honors student and wasn't used to condescension and constant monitoring. My mother was also trying to help me by meeting with the administration at the high school. She was trying to figure out a manageable schedule for me, while I was coping with numerous speech, occupational, and physical therapy sessions to obtain self-perceived normalcy.

After battles with the administration at my high school, I was finally allowed to use my extracurricular time spent at The Martinat Center (outpatient rehab) as my physical education requirement for two freshman semesters. There were always so many battles for such small things.

The physical therapist who worked with me at Martinat was named Annette. She was pretty, supportive, and friendly. She also made me work harder than I could ever remember working before. That's not really saying much when a person with short-term memory difficulties says it, though. She taught or reminded me how to walk well, run, and even swim again.

She asked if I remembered how to swim. I told her about working with a physical therapist at Myers Lake Rehab named Susie. The first time Susie took me swimming, I launched into the butterfly stroke, outpaced Susie, and slammed my head into the other side of the small pool.

Annette was mortified, knowing that another traumatic blow to my head might kill or damage me permanently. Obviously, that was not the case during in-patient rehab and I was fine... a little confused by what transpired, but basically fine. My mother, on the other hand, was stunned and perturbed by the pool collision. Annette used caution with me after hearing that story.

One especially tiring day at Martinat, I asked Annette why I looked so funny walking. I often watched myself in the mirror doing normal tasks (walking, talking, singing) to see if I resembled others who hadn't dealt with similar circumstances. Annette said that my gait was crooked because I was placing more weight and relying more on my right leg. The left side of my body had been numb for a period in the hospital, so I was thrusting the bulk of my body's weight onto my right leg when I walked. I don't remember what exercises she had me do to help strengthen my left side, but they worked. She also taught me to run, and I remember that day clearly and fondly. She said, "You're not ready. Your middle is frozen and your left side is still fairly numb."

"I'm going to run today," I said, completely ignoring her words. Sometimes it simply wasn't worth arguing with me, as I would unknowingly perseverate until I got my way. So Annette finally decided to help me instead of furthering the argument.

"Lift your left knee two inches higher," she said. She then instructed me to run with my hands loosely resting on the parallel bars. It worked and she led me outside, holding my hand as I ran. Annette and I ran all the way around the entire building! Running on grass was harder than running indoors; yet I didn't fall that day. Then we returned inside to face my nemesis, the dreaded stairstepper.

"I hate the stairstepper. I always fall. Why do I have to do it every day for five minutes?" I complained. Annette merely smiled and motioned for me to step on the ominous machine.

"And when I go home, I can't rest. I don't know why staying awake is important but it is. I have to study and study with mother. That's all I ever do. I take tests right after I study or I'll forget stuff. I make A's that way. And sometimes I watch TV but I don't like movies. I can't remember who did what. I like music. I am learning rap lyrics. They help me move my tongue. I want to talk faster and better. I sound like a robot, awful and slow. My words don't come out right. Music helps."

When my ranting was complete, Annette would just give me a hug. We would then move on to my next exercise where I would again complain about a new form of physical torture. (Today I only run in private. I only run on treadmills, preferably away from the public eye. I run a little jerky. Probably no one notices my gait irregularities but me).

During the day (either before or after Martinat), I'd attend high school for several hours and then return home for homebound tutoring sessions with Mrs. Gibson. Sometimes I would go to cheerleading practice; however, I couldn't take part in any stunts or anything that made the coaches uneasy. This was perfectly understandable. However, in later years, when I just wanted to practice cheers with my friends for camaraderie, this wasn't allowed, either.

The mirror in my home bedroom was removed when I smashed it after my release from the cheer squad. I know this because my chipped, antique mirror is now gone and is replaced by a flimsy, plastic one. I have physical clues like a new mirror to remind me of displaced memories.

Another clue is the eye patch in my dresser drawer. Wearing it made me feel like a pirate, and in Winston-Salem, there weren't many of those. God, I hated the eye patch. I kept trying to lose it, yet it kept coming back.

Other "fond memories?" In high school I was forced to face more surgeries that were wreck-related, but I was well enough at that point to *not* want to be readmitted to any medical facility. I developed granuloma anularae on my eyelids, an affliction noted often in the elderly, and probably acquired in the hospital. "But my face is the only normal part of me," I told Dr. Wright, plastic surgeon. He cut off the spreading bumpy places twice before a dermatologist reasoned that cortisone injections were more effective.

My diplopia was a huge problem, and I wouldn't wear eye patches in order to see single images. My parents took me to Dr. Weaver, a notable pediatric ophthalmologist. I asked him if corrective surgery could blind me, and he said, "Yes, it is delicate surgery which could blind both of your eyes." Great, I remember thinking. No wonder I delayed making a decision to undergo his knife.

"She will come to me," he told my mother. And Dr. Weaver was right... I would seek his help later on. But in the summer before my sophomore year, I was just beginning to realize how much I wanted to see better, move better, talk more fluently. I wanted to ride to and from school and social events without my parents taking me. Unfortunately, doctors said that even a minor blow to the head could kill or disable me, so friends were wary about allowing me to ride in their cars!

Abandonment by many of my former classmates—yes, I know I drooled and limped—hurt worse than the physical damages of my TBI. One day Zach said, "I picked Alex (a mutual friend) up for school today, and he came out of his door wearing a football helmet... I guess he didn't want me to give him a head injury, too!" I laughed. Zach felt terribly about the accident, and knowing this, his friends intentionally tried to offer me rides whenever possible. These rides helped me feel normal, and it doesn't matter why friends did it. Being with my classmates, even for short intervals, helped me recover emotionally.

Before summer '93 ended, I have "flicker memories" of my parents taking me out of town to practice being with other teens, in normal situations, like eating in restaurants. Oh, I hated restaurants. Forks and knives always seemed to fly out of my hands! I'm told I once put my face in a plate of mashed potatoes when I was frustrated with cutting—I believe this.

"Chicken sandwich," was my standard order, "and a straw with my coffee!" Waitresses brought the straws with the oddest looks.

I liked to play miniature golf left-handed, though it didn't always work. Some days both my hands trembled. Once I played with a dark-haired prep school boy, Douglas. We played a few holes and I told him my hand was injured. Then I missed the putt that would have beaten him. I not only missed it, but the ball sailed into a table of nearby adults. He looked at me strangely... So I threw my putter as hard as I could, right into the group that was staring at me. I mostly recall that shiny silver club, sailing through the air. No one was hurt, but I wouldn't have cared. I cared that I missed my winning putt.

"This was socially inappropriate behavior," my mother reminded me later. "The doctors all say you'll have trouble maintaining relationships while you act like this."

I wanted relationships badly.... But the world was out of my control.... What could I do? Maybe I needed a long-distance relationship.

"I'll write you," Douglas promised. I don't recall if he did or didn't. E-mail was not yet available. And I didn't really want to write letters. Controlling my body was difficult enough in the world of "normal" teenagers. Yet a few friends didn't mind my being different and slightly fragile.

Several days before my sophomore year began, my neighbor, Justin Brewster, and his girlfriend, Christy Sweat, offered to pick me up for school each day in exchange for a little gas money. They were friends of Zach's and were definitely braver than most. Why did they do this? I believe they wanted to help Zach by helping me. Also, Justin and I had been close friends. He knew I was sick of "mom," and I was.

8 Returning to a New Place

"If you are going through hell, keep going."
– Winston S. Churchill

My sophomore year of high school was my first full-time year post-TBI, and I try hard to recall it, but only images appear. I'd try to get dressed, only to have my mother argue about matching my shoes and socks. More arguing about my hiking boots looking strange, but they were the only footwear that supported my weak ankles. And riding to school, finally, with other teenagers.

Then getting to school, wondering if I was going to the right class each period. Falling down... hiding anywhere I could when I felt panicky. Trying to take a few notes with my left hand (which got easier with time). I simply couldn't concentrate on writing and listening to teachers simultaneously. I focused on drawing each letter of a word, rather than hearing discussions in class. Then I couldn't recall class lectures.

I did enjoy Spanish, which was somehow easy, remembered from Junior High classes. I enjoyed chorus where everyone was nice, but my favorite class was Honors English. Poetry was like music for me—short, easy, beautiful. But much of school was a nightmare: trying to get teachers to give me enough time to finish, to let me answer them before they interrupted me, getting enough nerve to raise my hand, and then give a wrong answer when the right one was still in my head. I know I hid in the bathroom often to calm down. Hiding in the bathroom relaxed me and helped me dodge people with walkie-talkies that tracked my movements through the high school. Clearly, liability issues plagued the administration, but I hated knowing staff members followed my every movement, every day, every minute.

Once I met a pregnant girl while escaping to the bathroom, a pretty brunette girl washing her hands. She obviously knew about me because she said, "Kelly, you and I are so much alike.... We are damaged goods. Sit with me at lunch if you need a friend." She made me feel somewhat better about my life. The father of her baby was now dating one of the freshmen, once my close buddy, who had stopped visiting me when I wasn't perfect and fun anymore. Well, as damaged goods, we were better off on our own.

Every morning I woke up worried about making a fool of myself at school. Every night I mentally reviewed the previous day, examining things I might have done wrong or assignments I forgot to do. Sleep was difficult.

And I tried to date in my sophomore year, but the whole thing was simply too difficult. I couldn't think of anything to say, and didn't want to kiss anyone. The idea of a tongue in my mouth made me want to vomit, and I just couldn't trust a strange guy with my huge problems. I had more important things to do, like making A's on tests and papers. An "A" meant more to me than an extended curfew. "A's" meant I was not diminished. They gave me a sense of control, of status. I didn't care how hard I had to work for that grade. One single "B" could literally make me throw up because I couldn't physically cry. Feelings of nausea replaced weeping, but maybe God wanted my tears.

Also in sophomore year, I met another "damaged" friend through Young Life of Winston-Salem. "Jake" had left his car running while he ran to get something. He forgot to set his parking brake, and the car rolled over a toddler; the child was dead and Jake was guilt-ridden like Zach. Maybe Jake was the first boy I ever wanted to kiss and I did, just once. He made me feel less alone somehow, although we only met occasionally. Between us there was too much pain in one room.

And that was the year when I lost everything every single day. I lost food, keys, purses, books, notes... my mother said she began taking a mental picture of me each time I left home so she could go and collect my things later. Thankfully, she also said, "It's just stuff... if we don't get it back, who cares?"

My sister Tyler also helped me to stop obsessing about what I couldn't do and could never remember. Tyler was away at college, but Wake Forest was nearby. No matter how busy she was, Tyler made time to help me with difficult Spanish homework. Once she wrote an entire poem in Spanish for me; however, cheating added to feelings of imperfection, so I avoided it. And Tyler understood. She knew I was trapped at home, and sometimes she let me stay in her dorm at Wake Forest.

Tyler was a Sigma Chi sweetheart, and her boyfriend didn't mind if I went to fraternity parties with them. Some Sigma Chi guys actually tried to pick me up, because with all the drinking and noise, they couldn't tell I was 15 and damaged. I realized then that boys don't much care about the little imperfections; they just want a pretty girl to dance or drink with. The Sigma Chi's gave me back a shred of self-esteem, but Tyler wouldn't leave me alone with them. She said, "There's nothing wrong with you that a drunken Sigma Chi will care about," and how right she was.

My sister was—and is—a wonderful, loyal, and very wise sister. Watching her life as an ACC cheerleader, a member of Kappa Kappa Gamma, President of Golden Key, Phi Beta Kappa, I began to long for college. But high school had to be endured first. Yet I was finally able to dream about a future, and stop wishing to die every hour of every day. Tyler gave me a dream.

My sister was probably the first person I consistently copied, physically. She looks like *Alice in Wonderland*, and even though a bit shy, Tyler always attracts attention with her bright inviting smile. I would close my door and stare in my bedroom mirror constantly. I copied Tyler's grins, frowns, raised eyebrows, posture, and gait. Maybe, I thought, people wouldn't focus on my slow speech if I could look like her. I wanted to force my face to have more expression, since my facial muscles didn't move on command. Doctors said my "affect" was somewhat paralyzed.

I loved movies with Reese Witherspoon. She was so bouncy and adorable in movies like *Legally Blonde*. I emulated her so much that I'm surprised no one noticed. Or maybe they did. Some people nicknamed me "Gidget," which I despised, although I had no concept of "Gidget" at that time. And I frequently rented the film *Dazed and Confused*. I enjoyed watching Matthew McConaughey and Ben Affleck, but I mainly wanted to copy the pouts of the high school girls they found attractive. My mirror was my own original therapy. It's funny, but when practicing facial expressions, I came up with some really scary faces I still use today. My father hates them! But most of life wasn't funny back then.

And I tried to relearn humor, which is hard for people recovering from TBI. The timing of a joke, I discovered, is more important than the material. Once in class, I made a hilarious joke about a map. The teacher pointed to Czechoslovakia, asked the class what country she was pointing to, and I yelled, "Kansas!", thinking that was funny. But no one even giggled. I looked around and waited... nope, not funny. Well, the shapes of the country and state were somewhat similar. Years later, I learned that teacher Mary Storch had warned students: "Anyone who laughs at Kelly—even once—gets an automatic F!!" I sure wish I'd known that then.

Often in school people would say, "Kelly, you look great, you're doing so well!" But I wasn't. Encouragement is one thing, but honesty has its merits. TBI taught me the value of the truth, even when it cuts. I could actually feel the lies of my classmates. Okay, so they didn't know what to say to me. But some friends were honest, as was my family. Even my father would say, "Go back and find some better shoes for that outfit... I hate the hiking boots with green socks." Nicole and Suzanne, Summit School friends, actually made tapes of my voice recorded by their message machines. They played them back for me to hear. I didn't recognize and loathed my slow, monotone speech, and of course this depressed and panicked me. But it also fired me up to speak faster and to vary my intonation. Finding truthful advocates is a large part of TBI recovery.

My world had simply changed too fast. My hobbies had disappeared—the art, the cheering, the horseback riding and soccer. I missed Chumley the horse, who "smacked" his lips only for me. I began to despise the telephone, which used to ring every five minutes when I was popular and healthy. Now it wouldn't ring for me most of the time. I stared at it a lot, and on the rare occasions, when the phone did ring, I couldn't think of things to say, or answer questions fast enough. I might say something stupid, or mean, or wrong. My mother helped a little by keeping a legal pad by the telephone. She wrote down "girl" things to talk about, and "guy" things. I think she sometimes enjoyed going back to high school mentally. I know she enjoyed keeping me "in style." She taught me to always wear black to avoid mismatches... black shoes, purse, and slacks. I do this today for the most part. But she couldn't talk on the phone for me.

She said people usually enjoy speaking about themselves. "See if you can get them talking about a personal topic or something." Tips like this lowered my anxiety. I couldn't remember the social "rules" everyone else seemed to know. The emotional stress of just one hour was greater than recurring physical pain.

The best therapy for me that fall of '93 came accidentally. A friend, Mrs. Mitchell, asked if her daughter Caroline could study for history tests with my mother, who was also a tutor. Both Caroline and I needed more review than average, and I pre-studied so I would look smart to her! Caroline was happy to come once a week to study, and was even more delighted when she began making A's in history.

She was the most beautiful girl in my class. With her car parked in front of my house, this history study group grew exponentially. That wasn't in the original plan, but it worked out really well. Other friends began asking if they could come and study before tests, and my mother began Xeroxing notes for each kid. These sessions were fun, and we started ordering pizzas and studying during the supper hour in order not to conflict with school activities. Before long we had ten or more in the group every week.

I think my mother was more than a little sneaky, as she figured the kids might as well meet on nights when I needed transport to school events. This way I didn't always have to call and beg for rides, which I found humiliating. Many history sessions ended just as Young Life meetings were beginning, so I had my pick of rides. It felt so good to be a part of my peer group again, even if the focus was studying the Fall of Rome.

My junior and senior years of high school were slightly easier for me than the first two, even though I went to bed each night wondering what vital information I'd forgotten from the previous day. But I did have a "life."

I became a bit cleverer about not losing my possessions. My female friends never wore purses and kept their driver's licenses in the pockets of jeans. Naturally I did this as well, and sometimes lost my license. This drove my mother crazy! She begged me to keep my vital things in one purse, especially my keys and license (but I refused for at least five years). So, I suggested getting duplicates of things. For example, every month or so I went to the DMV and said, "I've lost my license!" For ten dollars, I'd receive a duplicate that I kept in my glove compartment. I learned to keep copies of important things in convenient places. My mom and I were adapting to each other's needs. I began to be grateful for her tutorial help. In exchange for my cooperation and patience during excessive study, she let me shave my own legs despite the pools of blood I left in the bathtub. I preferred scars to assistance. The left hand switch continued to be difficult, but was improving.

One thing that really helped was a pool table in our den. I'd always played certain sports left-handed, and I was really proficient with pool. When I felt unsteady, I could lean against the table, then shoot. Pool was a social sport, and I felt comfortable inviting friends over to play. I could excel at, perhaps, at least one thing.

I also tried cooking, and even today dad tells me he *likes* blood in his tossed salad! My aunt LaLa, fortunately, started giving me kitchen gadgets that let me cut vegetables and not fingers. She bought me dishes and bowls made of plastic to make me feel less horrible about breaking things. I was awkward and clumsy—Hurray for Corelle and Tupperware!

In the fall of my junior year, I took guitar lessons from a boy named Mark. He attended a nearby high school, and I remember thinking he was very cute. My mother tells me I first met Mark at Young Life of Winston-Salem. It was the one place I met friends who didn't see me at my worst, undergoing the arduous tasks of the school day. And I loved to flirt with Mark, who was fairly tall with brown eyes and hair. I had a huge crush on him, but he somehow graciously said that he wasn't looking for a serious girlfriend. I don't remember being too upset about that, but Mark later informed me he had a very good friend who was interested in finding his "special someone." He said he would introduce me to "the nicest guy he knew" on a Young Life retreat we'd both be attending the following weekend.

I was excited about the winter retreat at Windy Gap, NC. However, I had numerous things to be fearful of. First of all was the packing. My parents often said the clothes I chose to wear seldom matched and were out of season. With my short-term memory problems, this situation would replay itself again and again. Thus, I required some serious assistance packing and putting together outfits to wear over the weekend.

I was concerned with being apart from my family for several days. The feeling wasn't homesickness, but it was close. My parents were the only people I knew I could trust and rely on 100% of the time. Other people took one look at me and assumed I was fine. I had no broken bones, wasn't blind, deaf or mute, and could hold a reasonably coherent conversation with a person on a one-on-one basis. When in group settings, I tended to tense up and hardly speak with anyone. I've heard people (mainly doctors) refer to TBI as the "invisible illness," because you can't simply take a look at people recovering from brain injuries and immediately see there is something wrong with them. You don't think to offer them appropriate aid. For instance, you wouldn't tell a blind man crossing the street to watch where he's going. This is the equivalent of telling a person with a traumatic brain injury to pay attention and speak rapidly.

Nevertheless, once we reached Windy Gap, it took me several hours to find and speak to Mark. He then found his friend, Lee, and formally introduced us. Lee and I had a wonderful time talking and walking around the campgrounds together. He asked if I wanted to go on a walk with him on one of the trails. I was extremely flattered that he wanted to spend time talking with me when there were so many more interesting people around to converse with. Without hesitation, I told Lee that I would like to walk with him in the mountains. As I was saying this, I was afraid that my poor walking skills due to my irregular gait would make me lose my balance or do something embarrassing. Also, I was concerned that Lee would go back to his friends after our walk and make fun of me. Taking a deep breath, I took Lee's hand and we began our walk around the outskirts of the campsite.

We came to a creek. Lee jumped from one rock to another until he had successfully crossed the water. However, my feet had not budged since he'd left. Lee, now on the far side, turned and looked inquisitively at me. Before I had the chance to explain my hesitancy, Lee jumped back to my side of the water, somehow understanding and empathizing with my difficulties. Lee put his arm around my waist, scooped me up and carried me across the creek. For an instant I was dumbfounded. Lee had known, without my telling him, exactly what I had needed and wanted. I was sure Mark had told him what he knew of my limitations; however, Mark hadn't known of my poor eyesight. Lee's intuition at the creek that day astounded me.

Lee quickly became my entire life. He made me feel normal, and didn't mind my idiosyncrasies, my stumbling, my odd behaviors. For instance, on our first date, I was supposed to meet him at a high school basketball game. I arrived very early because climbing bleachers was hard for me, and I didn't want people watching. I climbed high up, and remember watching Lee enter the gym, not seeing me at first. When he caught sight of me, he beckoned for me to come and sit with him. However, I didn't leave my seat until halftime. I couldn't climb through a jam-packed set of bleachers. I wondered, "Will he leave? Will he think I don't like him? If I try to descend and fall into the crowd, will people laugh?"

As ever, my smallest life decisions involved my TBI. I decided to stay seated until the crowd thinned. And he stayed. When I finally reached Lee, I explained to him my hesitancy in moving locations. My vision, when looking from either side to side or straight down, was terribly impaired. I had double vision at such angles. This was yet another thing I hated explaining to Lee. I had to remind him again of my many imperfections. Lee would simply nod with overwhelming concern. Later, he never minded tying my shoelaces for me, or driving me wherever I needed to go. He relieved me of the daily anxiety of catching rides with classmates, for I still hated to ride with family members. Teens don't want to be with parents much, and I despised having family drive me to sporting events, parties, and the mall. In brief, Lee made me seem more normal than I would have seemed otherwise. He also helped me academically.

In history class, I remember having to break up into groups and do a project on an assigned decade in American history. My group chose the '50s, with poodle skirts, '57 Chevys, and "Fonzie" guys with sideburns and greasy hair. I met Jeff in that history group. Jeff was and is a good and true friend who helped me tremendously throughout high school and beyond. He needed a reasonably good grade on this project, and I always needed an A. So we all worked diligently while trying to come up with something that would make our decade stand out.

I talked with Lee about the situation, and he had an absolutely perfect idea. If I could get school permission, Lee would drive his father's red '57 Chevy to the history building, and I could walk my class out to look at it as the finale of our presentation. Lee agreed to be in costume, wearing a leather jacket and jeans.

The day of the presentation arrived and everyone in the group was dressed appropriately in 1950s attire, girls in sweater sets and pleated skirts and boys in jeans and white T-shirts. Each person described an aspect (music, home life, television) of the decade. When we were almost finished, I opened the door in the back of the classroom and Lee roared to a stop in his '57 Chevy. My group and I led the class out of the door and straight to the parking lot. I then informed the class that in the 1950s, this was "the coolest" means of transportation. I opened the passenger's side door and jumped in beside him. Lee revved the enormously loud engine and we drove away (around the block and then back to school). My group made an A on our project.

I mention this because it was a collaboration, an alliance. I often developed a fondness for particular, multisyllabic words because I'd discovered that big words were easier for me to spell than small ones, and because people thought I was still smart when I used them. The history project was an alliance, and I realized I was not alone in my struggle for academic normalcy.

Another word I became intrigued with was *networking*. If I really needed something, I could network! I could form an alliance. Before this project I had pinned my hopes for help at school on the "higher ups." Now I pinned hopes on Lee and various classmates, instead of relying on friends in high places like the school's administration. I realized the value of friends in low places, as they came in handy and were more reliable.

On my 17th birthday, Lee gave me my favorite kind of present, an experience. He gave me ponies and rainbows. We went to his family's beach house, took a ferry to Shackleford Banks, and watched the wild ponies running. It drizzled and a huge rainbow appeared. It was then I realized how special and how real the bond Lee and I had created was. Today I still occasionally lose "things." I dislike valuable gifts, and prefer to do something special when I celebrate. My mother said I always had this preference, showing me a poem I wrote (but don't remember writing) at age 9:

Tomorrow is my birthday
But don't give me CDs
Just give me an experience
I want some memories.

I had told my mother, "I only need one true friend to be happy." Now I had that, and was indeed happier. But I would learn that one friend, while excellent, is not enough. The last two years of high school were far better than the first two, but I still suffered from a dire girlfriend shortage. Girls didn't accept my altered behaviors as easily as boys. Boys looked at me and saw a cute girl who was recovering from an accident. Girls saw a different Kelly, an inferior Kelly, an embarrassment at times.

Every day as a precedent-setting student with TBI classification at Reynolds High School was difficult, but sporadic events stand out as being especially helpful. In my junior year I begged to be the manager of the cheerleading squad, which meant I could attend pre-game dinners with my former squad, and then ride in the bus to games. The principal agreed. I've learned since that the cheer coaches really didn't want to be responsible for me, but my mother pushed the issue, and my principal finally agreed. Every ride helped. I still couldn't see well enough to drive alone to distant games.

But I could see well enough to attend movies. The movie I most remember from high school is *Rudy*, the true-life story of Daniel E. "Rudy" Ruettiger, a young steel mill worker, who desperately wanted to play football for Notre Dame. From time to time, I met with a wonderful neuropsychologist, Dr. Frank B. Wood. I really liked Dr. Wood, but I think I worried him one day when he asked me how I felt about God. I answered, "There are two things I'm sure of—there is a God, and I'm not Him!" I don't think Dr. Wood had seen the film. He informed my parents that my views on religion were a bit unusual. He later wrote my parents that my responses that day had been rather sardonic. And Dr. Wood was surely right. However, he lifted my spirits; he told me I might, with the right credentials, be able to perform educational testing someday.

The second movie I recall is *Forrest Gump*. Ironically, I wasn't particularly affected by this disabled man's ability to pursue success. I simply enjoyed learning via film all the history Forrest covered—the "hippy" era, Civil Rights protests, and the Vietnam War. Movies helped me recover lost patches of history classes, or books I had read and forgotten. I really needed better vision to read more books unassisted.

As my junior year drew to a close, Lee said, "Kelly, think of all the things we could do if you had eye surgery. We could play tennis and golf so much easier." I eventually consented and went to Dr. Grey Weaver. Like he'd once predicted, I asked the doctor for corrective eye surgery despite my nervousness. The muscles behind my eyes had been severely stretched by the blow to my head, and the surgery involved cutting directly into the whites of both eyes to repair the damage behind.

I didn't want both of my eyes worked on at the same time. However, Dr. Weaver explained that by doing both at once, a balance could be obtained between the eyes, allowing me to see evenly once more. This was the man who didn't know I tried to cheat on his previous eye tests. Later I somehow memorized one eye chart before taking an exam to pass my driving test. Had my brain willed my short-term memory to temporarily overcome my handicaps to obtain my driver's permit?

Much more importantly, could I risk never being able to drive or to see again? I already had enough problems!

But my parents and Lee kept encouraging me, and the day came for surgery. One of my clearest memories of that time is waiting with my mother and Lee to be rolled into surgery. A nurse with an empty stretcher passed by us.

"There goes another one that didn't make it!" Lee said, smiling. We all cracked up, and the laughter helped as they rolled me away. Afterwards, I was released with no nights in the hospital, which turned out to be a big mistake. My eyes were totally red and I looked like a vampire. And the pain was tremendous. I was very nauseated, but was told not to throw up or my stitches could break, requiring further surgery.

My parents, LaLa, and Lee stayed up with me all night, taking turns placing ice packs on my eyes every 20 minutes. Today I have 20/20 vision. This has released me from my geographic trap somewhat, and I can drive to work and important places on my own. I still do not drive on highways where multiple cars can drive past me on either side. My peripheral vision remains minimally impaired.

But driving gave me a new problem to solve. I had to remember where to go! I had dated a little before Lee carried me over a creek, but most boys refused to put up with my slow speech, and my inability to drive and drink. Lee's house was about four miles from mine, with numerous twists and turns, yet I had renewed energy with my eyes coming into focus. My father promised to drive to Lee's house as often as I wished, with me following in my own car. Eventually, he thought, my kinesthetic memory would kick in and I could drive the path on my own.

Well, after nine trips I was still getting lost. I replayed the route in my head, and tried yet one more time, and I got there. It took me ten times, yet that was better than the 51 times it took me to jump a rope, better than the 24 times it took for me to memorize a certain geometry theorem. Maybe my ability to memorize new material was getting better. Maybe I was finally improving!

Lee also gave me self-confidence at a time when I sorely needed it. With my new and positive outlook on life, I suddenly began to enter into social settings and engage in conversations with friends without nerves interfering. Lee's friends (mostly guys) were extremely nice to me, and for the first time in a long time, I began to feel like I belonged again. My new friends accepted me for who and what I was. They enjoyed my company and even laughed at some of my jokes.

When Lee graduated from high school and chose to attend Wake Forest University in Winston-Salem, I was elated. I felt very special being a senior in high school and dating a man in college. Before entering Wake, Lee had to purchase a ThinkPad laptop computer to accompany him to each class. Wake Forest University was the first in the nation to require an incoming class to own identical laptop computers, and Lee was in the experimental group. His class notes and assignments would be available to him online via e-mail and on the teacher's homepage. Lee found out that he was required to take a class in how to use this laptop. I don't think he was excited about adding another academic requirement to his already full schedule, but he didn't have a choice. I remember feeling great sympathy toward Lee, as he was nervous embarking on his collegiate career. However, his acquisition of a laptop at the beginning of the year turned out to be a hidden blessing for me, as Lee taught me most of what he learned in each computer class.

Lee left me with total confidence on the computer. My comfort level with programs like Word, PowerPoint, and Excel grew significantly. I was also realizing that while I couldn't write neatly or with a great amount of speed, I could type. When I had attended the private Summit School through 8th grade, I took numerous classes involving computers. At that time, the Internet was mainly utilized by the government. Computers used in classrooms were equipped with MS-DOS, which was considered advanced at the time. Following the accident, doctors kept informing my parents that I would be able to relearn information I had acquired prior to my TBI, more easily than totally new information. Also, my mother said that when I first returned from Myers Lake Rehab, the first thing I did when I walked in the back door was to sit down and switch on my family's Apple 2-E computer.

So in time and with weeks of practice, my typing skills increased exponentially (reaching approximately 18-20 words per minute), coinciding with the emergence of the Internet and the global integration of the computer. As I became more technologically advanced, people stopped noticing my hand tremors. This was a welcome change for me.

Lee also attempted to teach me (or help me relearn) how to play tennis with double vision. Tennis was tricky for me, as I saw two yellow balls coming at me instead of one. I would close my eyes just before impact and aim somewhere in between the two. Interestingly, this strategy was successful more often than not! Lee would also kick soccer balls with me and go hiking. He even tried to teach me how to drive his stick shift car, a truly disastrous action which left his car's transmission somewhere on the road behind us.

The most important thing Lee did for my recovery was to convince me to have surgery on my eyes. Today I am no longer confused by viewing the world in duplicate. If I happen to see two of an object, I'm now assured that there actually is a pair of something in front of me; however, I still can't seem to get the hang of tennis with only one ball to aim for. Lee was a great blessing for both me and my family. Anyone with TBI definitely needs and deserves a Lee in their life. I must have realized his devotion at the time because my journal in 12th-grade English records a rhyming couplet I don't remember writing:

He found me when my heart and eyes were closed
And took me past the limits I supposed.

Or maybe the most important thing he did was to love me as I was.

9 College Bound (1996)

"What you hope for, you also fear."

– Alice Walker

The summer after my senior year was, I guess, pretty typical. I was very happy to finally leave Reynolds High School. While Reynolds had done a few good things for me, it had done some pretty awful (not to mention demoralizing) things as well. The scales kept swinging—I blessed the math teachers who reinforced my memories with two consecutive algebra classes (the second as a study hall) —I cursed those who refused to allow me to type as required by my IEP. I loved Ms. Oakley and Ms. Powers for planning graduation so "Bouldin" sat at the bottom of the bleachers. I had nightmares about office staff slamming me down into chairs. How could college be worse?

I had recently made up my mind not to attend college at Elon University or N.C. State (where I was accepted), fearing that I honestly didn't want to be that far away from my parents or my boyfriend Lee. I decided to attend Salem College located in the restoration village of Old Salem, Winston-Salem. At the time I rationalized that I needed to be close to my doctors at Baptist Hospital, and there was a little truth in that.

Before making a final decision, I called many admissions counselors at North Carolina colleges and universities, asking, "Do you have any programs to assist students with TBI?"

Over a dozen persons answered, "What is TBI?" However, one faculty member at Salem College did have experience working with the brain-injured. Such knowledge was a plus for this fine liberal arts college, the first to educate women in America. So during my senior high school year, in March of '93, I attended an "overnight" at Salem College to fully experience what life on the collegiate level was like.

At the overnight I met a lovely, dynamic girl named Jennifer, and we became fast friends. By the end of the evening we agreed to be roommates the following year. I left the dorm feeling like I had a best friend to share all the exciting adventures college life had in store for me.

I telephoned Jennifer a week or two later to discuss our room layout for the freshman year, and she said she'd decided to attend Appalachian State University instead of Salem. I was devastated. I had built the next four years of my life at Salem so far up that it made me crazy to watch as it all fell tragically to the ground. Actually, someone changing their mind about where to attend college is quite normal; however, I feared that this setback might stop my positive flow of pre-college adrenaline.

I remember going to Salem's orientation in late August of 1996 and feeling a strange mixture of being excited, scared, sad, and impatient. I was definitely impatient for another chapter in my life, and for this chapter to be a positive one. I wasn't thinking at all about academics. My thoughts were consumed by the social situations which I feared I wasn't prepared to enter. I was right.

College was scary. As in high school, I kept forgetting where to go to class, who my teacher was, and where I put my schedule. I threw up a lot due to nerves in the first three weeks. I continued to have difficulty finding everything from my dorm room to the correct classrooms.

The registrar's office became my initial stop each morning before I began my academic schedule. The registrar was an older woman somewhat hard of hearing. She smelled faintly of mothballs. I would walk into the office and tell her, "I need another copy of my class schedule." She would ask me why I needed another copy, and I would have to go into the same reason or story that I'd probably given her the day before and perhaps the day before that, and so on. Honestly, if I'd been calm and not nervous about my situation, I could've remembered my schedule and the beginning and ending times for all of my classes.

Eventually, the woman with gray hair gave me another copy of the schedule, telling me not to lose it, as if that was anything I had control over or would even remember her telling me after several minutes had passed. Nonetheless, I had my schedule in hand and was off to my classes.

In English classes I felt moderately capable. Even though I had lost my ability to skillfully draw, I was still able to paint images in my mind with words. If given ample time, I would often use various literary conventions such as alliteration or assonance to tell of a feeling or thought. I could at least write a page during an hour-long class, provided I could use a laptop. On bad days, I forgot my laptop.

I vaguely remember that in each class, I always tried to contribute at least something to discussions. Usually what I said was correct and made sense. Each of these small contributions was an enormous social victory for me, but with stresses similar to those endured in high school, I began wanting to leave college. My teachers never gave me enough time to say what I meant, just like in high school. I found it difficult to sleep. I needed help. I just wasn't sure what kind... again, I thought I should have died in '93.

My mother once said that when I'd been at Salem College for two weeks, she received a call from the college president. She said, "I'm afraid Salem doesn't have what Kelly needs to be successful."

My mother replied, "It clearly does," as she was a '72 graduate of Salem College. My mother explained that my initial advisor had lost my medical file which explained my special needs. The advisor had also failed to give teachers pertinent data, and ignored promises regarding note takers and other accommodations. The president asked, "What exactly *does* Kelly need?"

My mother replied, "She needs two things. My daughter needs a friend as an advisor, and a Xerox machine to copy the daily notes taken by friends."

"That's all? You're sure?"

"Yes." The president then initiated a 3-way call with the advisor, who argued with my mother until the president ordered her to hang up. I was given a new advisor the following day. Life improved.

Academically, life was hard for a while. I made sure to take each instructor my own personal file of "crash data" for teachers unacquainted with TBI. Dorm life was another hardship, although I did manage to have a little fun. My roommate, Haley, was very friendly, blonde, and petite. The summer before entering Salem, we talked on the telephone and planned our room bedding and colors. We chose matching purple comforters with white flowers on them. I don't really remember my first days of school. I guess fear and anxiety clouded every experience, which might have been a blessing. That is one very important thing I learned a bit later about my new self. People who have suffered a severe brain injury don't often deal well with change. We like patterns and schedules and consistency. Thus, I didn't handle moving into a dorm, eating in a new cafeteria, attending new classes in new classrooms with new teachers, etc. at all well. Everything in my world had suddenly changed and I had no control over it. I couldn't even cry over my loss of stability.

Still, the beginning of college was more positive than negative. I invited a group of girls from my dorm over to my parents' house for a home-cooked meal, and everyone had a wonderful time. As the semester progressed, I must have started acting differently because the girls who were initially my friends began to act strangely around me. The girls would avoid me when talking about boys or clothes, and they never seemed to want me around. I remember pondering what I might have said or done to turn these friendships so far around. The only thing I didn't consider was the way I was interpreting the behavior of these girls. If my body was broken by my accident, then my mental composure was probably a little shaken as well. But I didn't consider that as a likely possibility. All of a sudden, the familiar feeling returned. I was alone again, but this time I was without my parents and I was afraid.

My academic schedule for the initial semester at Salem was a full load or four courses (including the college math course I passed over the summer). My parents and doctors didn't think it was wise for me to sign up for more than three courses in my first semester because they knew it would be too much emotional strain for me.

I remember entering my first class. I walked in and about 8–10 other girls stared back at me. A few smiled and some whispered to one another. The teacher pointed to a desk and I quickly sat down. As the class began, the teacher went around the classroom in a circle, calling on different students. She wanted each girl to tell the class her name, where she was from, and one interesting fact about herself. My turn arrived and I told everyone my name and one interesting fact.

"Hi, everyone. My name is Kelly Bouldin and I'm double-jointed in my hips and arms!" I said with a huge smile.

When prompted by the teacher, I added that I was from Winston-Salem originally. Most people said something about their pet at home or about an award they won in high school as their interesting fact. I didn't realize how strange my fact was until a few minutes after the introductory exercise concluded. I was worried the rest of the class would think I was weird or different, but when the session was over, several of the girls spoke to me. *Maybe being myself wasn't such a bad thing after all.*

After the first-day introductions ended and nightly homework began, I realized that I had no confidence whatsoever in completing assignments. I called my mother, who was my academic coach through high school. She asked me to calm down and to find my college advisor the next day. Nan Tilley was my advisor and helped me often. I had changed advisors when the special education liaison lost my records. I was afraid of that woman's harsh manner, and Ms. Tilley was the warm and fuzzy faculty friend I needed.

10 Psyched Out

"Sometimes it's the smallest decisions that can change your life forever."

- Keri Russell

I'm not sure how my parents found Dr. James Mattox, but I now realize that I owe my life to him. When my mother first suggested I accompany her to a psychiatrist back in high school, I said "No!" I felt that I was perfect and in no need of psychiatry. The world was broken, and I was somehow the only one who could see that.

Years later, when I was at Salem College, my mother said that Dr. Mattox could perhaps prescribe a medication that might assist me in managing my fluctuating anxiety levels. Even though I was mentally broken and lost in my mind, I knew I needed help. When I first met Dr. Mattox (Jimmy), I shook his hand and told him that I didn't want to be there. I didn't need some strange man asking me questions about my personal life, and the last thing I was in the mood to do was discuss my accident.

Before attending the session, my mother said the doctor already knew the details of the wreck, and that she would do most of the talking, as if I wasn't aware of that before she told me. I love my mother, but she can talk without taking a breath for hours. As my father says, my mother talks so much she gets herself into trouble. Even though her constant chatter was enough to push me toward insanity at times, I loved listening to her if it wasn't about school.

Therefore, I wasn't at all concerned that she would remain silent while I was divulging my innermost thoughts and feelings to the doctor, no matter how persistent he was. So the talking began. We went over the car crash, the TBI, my social ineptitude, the struggles I had been through and was currently facing, etc. I talked until my throat begged for silence, aching with a dull scratchy throb. When I finally finished my lengthy oration with only a few interruptions from my mother, Dr. Mattox asked me the usual questions I'd mentally been preparing for:

"What do you remember about the time you spent in the hospital?"

"Do you remember anything while you were in coma?"

Then he hit me with a question I hadn't heard before: "How did it make you feel when your friends abandoned you?" I had to stop and think. I knew I didn't appreciate being avoided and left alone during my free time, which I didn't really have much of anyway, but no one had ever asked me how I'd felt before.

I answered him quietly. "I don't know. I guess it made me feel pretty bad... I mean hurt."

After answering that key question, I began to realize that Dr. Mattox got it. Throughout the rest of our conversation, we exchanged questions and answers effortlessly. If my mother was in the room during that time, I wasn't aware of her. The all-encompassing feeling of a mutually meaningful dialogue overwhelmed me. Here I was, talking to a complete stranger (or at least he had been several minutes before) about my life, including all of my recent hindrances. Why couldn't the girls in my dorm be easy to talk with? In later years, I would learn that my fear of rejection impeded my social exchanges. I also struggled with receptive and expressive aphasia, or difficulty processing things said to me, coupled with similar difficulties speaking fluidly to others.

When Jimmy and I finished our conversation, I felt like the world was lifted off of my shaky shoulders. Even though I had truly needed and enjoyed our meeting, I was exhausted. The one other thing the meeting had made crystal clear was the fact that I was depressed... shocker! Of course I was depressed. I had lost many friends, my ability to speak at an appropriate speed and with clarity, physical abilities to play my favorite sports like horseback riding and others. I always had low self-esteem problems, and my accident only added to them. That day Dr. Mattox prescribed the antidepressant Zoloft for me. A miracle occurred. My life or my sanity had suddenly been handed back to me in the form of a tiny pill.

I followed my mother back to her house and took a nap on my favorite green love seat in our small den. My parents' house is two stories and is painted white with dark green shutters. It sits on a corner lot in the middle of a prestigious neighborhood, and the people who live there won't let you forget it. If you haven't noticed, I have a bad tendency of jumping from topic to topic. I will do my best to stop and try not to confuse you further.

After my initial visit to my new doctor, I would only see him in times of great trauma in my life. Several times this trauma was due to a boyfriend break up, but that is for another chapter. The Zoloft Dr. Mattox prescribed for me was a true lifesaver. My daily feelings of rejection and sadness seemed to vanish shortly after taking that little yellow pill. I didn't experience any of the negative side effects associated with Zoloft. Actually, I may have felt a little invincible for a few years after beginning the medication, but if you know what the side effects of any medication are, you can watch out for them.

My mother said that my doctors didn't want me taking any kind of medication during the first three years or so following my accident because they feared it would slow the healing rate of my brain.

"You don't want to anesthetize a waking brain," some said. Doctors had also informed my parents that what I did not regain within the first two to five years following my accident, I probably never would. The previous information was false in my case, as I now watch my right hand stabilize more and more each day. The Zoloft did help me feel a little more comfortable entering into conversations both inside and outside of the classroom. I no longer analyzed probable responses to questions I had never been confident enough to ask in the first place.

The brightest spot in what seemed to me like an ever-changing future was Lee. He seemed to understand what I was going through and the hardships I was facing in college. When Lee was with me at the dorm, I felt strangely "normal." The only problem with that was that he couldn't be with me 24/7. After the first few months of college, I was closer than usual to breaking. Recurring thoughts of suicide invaded my mind, and I knew I needed a different kind of help. If "Uncle Jimmy" hadn't prescribed antidepressants, I doubt I would be here today.

Post-Zoloft, my depression and emotions regarding life in college, were much more stable. I remember telling my mother that with Zoloft, I felt like myself again. Lee could also see an immediate difference in my personality and was very pleased with my new sense of self. I was hoping my new pill would magically eradicate my social dilemmas; however, that was a bit much to ask for.

When I returned to Babcock (my dormitory) one evening, the freshman class was gathered in the basement for a meeting. I had known about this gathering but had forgotten. Luckily I was able to say a quick goodbye to Lee and race downstairs to take part in the conference. I glanced around the room and quickly sat down beside my roommate, Haley. She was almost a foot shorter than I with long, straight, blonde hair. I had always been envious of any girl possessing fair hair, and had been highlighting my hair ever since I turned 13. (One of my worst problems in rehab, for me, was a return to mousy brown—no time for hair frostings there). At any rate, Haley didn't say much at first, but as people got to know her, she would quickly let them into her cheerful, self-confident world. I was very happy this adorable girl was my roommate, as we seemed to have much in common.

As our class meeting progressed, I learned that we needed to elect a class president, vice president, and treasurer. In order for everyone in the room to learn my face and name, I thought that I should run for something. Haley thought it was a good idea as well. I decided to run for vice president. I figured that as the vice president, I wouldn't have to make any difficult decisions. I would merely assist the class president with whatever she was doing, and delegate the rest of my duties.

Each of the candidates stood up and gave the audience some interesting facts about themselves and what they would do if elected to class office. When my turn came, I stood up and introduced myself as everyone had done before me. I could feel the eyes of strangers glaring my way, but when I was finished, everyone smiled and clapped. I wish I remembered what I said precisely, but I know I felt extremely pleased (even a little smug) about the new person I was becoming at Salem.

As high as I was at that point, when the election results were read, I was as equally low. I lost. I just couldn't seem to get a break. When I returned with Haley back to our room, she said a few consoling words and then went to a new friend's room. I was so jealous of Haley's ability to make friends. I wanted more than anything to make new and lifelong friendships with the people in my dorm. However, when I tried, the outcome was sadly different. I couldn't figure out why other girls, who had seemed to like me at the beginning of college, suddenly began avoiding me in the hallways. I always tried to be friendly, but the girls in my dorm seemed to be able to sense that I was somehow different than they were.

Looking back on those days with my current knowledge of personality alterations associated with traumatic brain injury, I still cannot see why those girls were so unfriendly and, at times, rude to me.

I agree with my late grandmother's philosophy that "there is never an excuse for rude behavior." Maybe I seemed rude by not talking as much as others, but I stayed silent often, rather than confuse my thoughts and words. I also found that my slower speech bored people, and a mere few allowed me to finish my thoughts without interruption.

As the days passed, I learned to cope with my dorm-mates. Basically avoiding them and keeping to myself as much as possible seemed to be my best course of action. Haley was a good roommate, but even she turned out to be a little worldlier than I. Having been in a car wreck my first few days of high school, I had missed all of what was encompassed in a "normal," 1990s high school experience. Drugs and sex had seemed like mere annoyances in high school, but such things had rapidly permeated the centuries-old walls of Salem College.

One day I was astounded to enter my dorm room and find a friend's ex-boyfriend sitting on my carpet making marijuana cigarettes. Today this would not shock me, but then, I was so far beyond *freaked out* by this experience that I drove home and stayed with my parents that night. I was—perhaps—your stereotypical freshman, being both naïve and frightened. Was my reaction to what occurred in my dorm room an unusual reaction brought on by my head injury, or had I reacted in a normal, age-appropriate fashion? As I grew up for the second time, I would ask myself that very question many times. Was I experiencing the normal feelings of a young adult, or were the feelings unique to me, recovering from TBI? In the end, the question didn't matter, because either way I had to deal with my feelings. I became truly great at rationalizing things, but perhaps we all do.

Now that I was beginning to question my position in the universe, my thoughts turned to religion. I couldn't help it—every day I heard the quarter-hour chimes of Home Moravian Church in Old Salem.

I thought if there is a God, as I was taught to believe, why had the accident happened? I mean, I was a relatively "good girl." Why then did I encounter such a horrific thing? If God is up on His cloud in the proverbial heavens, why then did He not somehow intervene on my behalf? I was completely certain that if the Almighty was able to intervene and alter situational outcomes, then I had a problem viewing Him as my Savior. For all I knew, I hadn't been saved.

When I was in a coma, I didn't remember anything. Coma was similar to going to sleep at night and waking up the next morning, but the next morning, I couldn't walk, talk, or even sit up without assistance. How could years of social and mental torture, coupled with a newly acquired learning disability and years of physical therapy, equal my salvation? If God thought that one up, then He obviously needed to keep on thinking.

I discussed religion with my parents, friends, and faculty. I decided that the only way I could believe in the Lord again would be if He were incapable of changing anything on the Earth. When I now think about God, it still helps to imagine Him on or at least amongst the clouds. When there is any kind of calamity, I believe the Lord (or at least the one I follow) always cries with and for the injured.... but He can't intervene. Keeping these and other beliefs close to my heart and mind helps me maintain some kind of a religious view in my life. My grandmother once said, "It is not difficult to believe in something greater than yourself." But some days, I think she was wrong.

I remember one Sunday, about eleven months after my accident, I felt compelled to go to my church, Home Moravian Church. I woke my mother up and told her to get dressed fast. Somewhat startled, she agreed to go with me. She was startled because I'd refused to go before, yet on that morning, I felt compelled to attend. Toward the end of that day's sermon, the minister read the verse Romans 8:18. It was the verse that Britt Armfield had written in a letter to my parents shortly after my accident. Having Romans 8:18 read in a service where I was present was a very surreal experience. It was almost as if Britt himself was telling me to hold on, keep working, and my life would eventually improve. My mother and others used to ask me why I worked so compulsively hard to regain everything I had lost. The answer to that is simple. I wanted it all. Yet I wouldn't have worked as hard as I did if I had known how long it would take for me to get "everything" back. In retrospect, I am thankful to my non-intervening God that I didn't know.

Today, I definitely believe in something. Call it God, Buddha, whatever. I'm sure beyond a shadow of a doubt, that there is Something out there, a lot more powerful than I. No longer am I concerned with wondering exactly who or what God is, though. I figure that, in time, I'll find out.

11 Speaking and Acting Out

"If you don't take risks, you'll have a wasted soul."
- Drew Barrymore

So college went on for me. My freshman year was difficult, but bearable. My mother never relented in her desire to bring me out of denial, which she felt was a terrible problem for me. Yes, I did attempt much more than I was capable of. Yes, I often denied I was different or slow or incapable of doing what others could do. But she often tested my limits. One notable time was when she said that Dr. Sandra Adams of Summit School, the private school I attended through 8th grade, wanted me to give a talk to her junior high students. Evidently some of them were not being nice to each other, and she thought that hearing from me might make them kinder in spirit. I was so scared to talk on stage. I was mostly afraid that I would forget things and make mistakes. My mother said we could do this together, and I wanted to help individuals with traumatic brain injury in the future. I could do this. I wrote my first public address on TBI, comforted by the fact that my mother would participate, and knowing my audience needed simple speech and some plain hard facts about friendship and its value.

My speech was well received and was published in the *Summit Echoes*, a school magazine which was mailed to alumnae. This upset me at first because I hadn't prepared myself for such a public display of my disabilities and problems. Today I'm glad many people read my words. The openness helped me to confront more problems to come, like deciding on a course of study.

In choosing a college major, I had to be extremely selective. Once I considered art, yet my bilateral hand impairment pretty much ruled out painting and sculpture. In high school, I had tried photography, but kept forgetting which lens to use, which setting to adjust. Initially I ruled out education because I was sick of the world of academia. I considered Spanish, but knew I had a tendency to forget vocabulary words. So, my mother and I made a pot of fresh coffee, and chose a more practical route.

We consulted yearbook pictures of Salem College faculty and narrowed my major choices by counting the number of male teachers in each field. Personal evidence had taught me in high school that males were more sympathetic to girls with disabilities. This, of course, is my opinion. I discovered that a bachelor's in Business or Communication would yield me the highest percentage of male professors. Ever since changing from the right to left hand, I occasionally wrote number reversals, and my advisor liked the idea of placing me in front of a camera. Therefore, Communication it was!

Fortunately, we lived only a few hours from Wilmington, NC, where the teen saga *Dawson's Creek* was being filmed. The teen soap opera also piqued my interest in the film world, so I faxed my photograph to a casting agency on the coast. They hired me, and I occasionally worked as an extra on this coastal set. I was proud to do this on my own with no help from my family... except for the driving part. Yes, I met Katie Holmes. No, she won't remember me. I did, however, discover that those in the acting and production world are very tolerant of differences. I felt at home with entertainers, then and now.

Ultimately, Communication with emphasis in Broadcasting and Production was a suitable major for me. I learned much about computers that I never knew, which added to a broad base I had never forgotten post-TBI. (Those Apple 2-E games like "Frogger" were not erased from memory, short- or long-term.)

Competent in my "Com" courses, I enjoyed college more. The environment did, over time, give me back an element of normalcy and simple fun. I finally lived in a world where nobody knew about my handicaps unless I showed them or told them.

One night I went to a frat party at Wake Forest University, and a cute guy named Parker asked me to dance. Later he walked me back to my car. I was holding a drink he probably thought was beer (it was Coke), and he tried too hard to convince me to go up to his room and hang out for a while. I tried to tell him that for me, "casual sex" is an oxymoron.

He either wouldn't listen, or I was talking too slowly. Anyway, I just dumped my drink on his head and left as he cursed. And isn't that a fairly normal thing to do? Maybe, but my inability to communicate verbally makes me feel guilty, anxious, different. On good days I am queen of the one-liner, able to conjure up a quick and snappy comeback remark for anyone. On other days the words stay in my head and swirl around, unspoken and toxic.

I also remember driving to my parents' house and openly complaining about the caliber of men I was meeting at frat parties and bars. While I was talking, my father left the room. He returned after about fifteen minutes and handed me a typed list:

Eight Rules for Dating
(by my father, Bob Bouldin)

1. Don't date anyone that doesn't have a full-time, acceptable job.
2. Don't date anyone you meet in a bar.
3. Don't live with anyone until you are married.
4. Don't discuss money with dates.
5. Smile often.
6. Be mysterious and aloof some of the time.
7. Be a lady—don't act silly, crude, or immature.
8. Don't be too outspoken.

Great. I was now accepting dating advice from my father, but at least I knew he meant well. I eventually returned to my dorm where I felt much more normal commiserating with friends about guy problems. We talked about boys and academic issues for hours. We also shared a growing obsession with the Internet, still new to most of us then. My father was the victim of my first attempt to shop online in the '90s. So he perhaps earned the right to give me dating advice.

I was learning that airline tickets could be purchased on the Internet. Wow... a way out of my narrow geographic walls. If I could fly someplace, I wouldn't need to drive and endanger people. So I bought a ticket to Myrtle Beach, SC, to visit a cute blonde boy I met at a party. Or I thought I bought the ticket.

My last trip on an airplane had been to the Bahamas with Tyler and my parents. My father had paper tickets sent to our home via what we now call "snail mail." Anyway, with directions from a friend, I called up Expedia, typed in a VISA number (don't know whose), as well as my dates of travel.

"How do I get this ticket?" I asked the friend.

"It's an e-ticket," she said, "and you just check in at the airport in Raleigh."

When the Friday arrived for my big date on the coast, I couldn't find a friend to drive me to the airport, so I called my father. He was angry but unwilling to sacrifice the cost of the ticket, so he drove me to Raleigh that day. But the e-ticket wasn't there for me. I hadn't pushed the "send" button and had no flight. So my sweet father drove me all the way to Myrtle Beach and then made the five-hour trip back to Winston. Yes, he had the right to give me lists when choosing guys, and the right to far more. I don't recall how I got home from that weekend journey. I was clearly not stable in the collegiate world, Internet world, or in any world at all. Being stable in college is hard for anyone with or without a handicap.

But then, like a gift from whatever gods exist, there was Amanda Waugh. I doubt if I would have graduated from college without meeting her. Having decided to make my disabilities public, and to help those suffering from TBI whenever a chance came about, I accepted an invitation from a Salem professor to speak to his biology class when the group was analyzing the brain and its functions. I was (and still am) always nervous in front of a group. I will never speak as rapidly as I did pre-wreck, and at age twenty, my fears of public speaking were tremendous.

Dr. Nolgren simply said to answer group questions, although I did give a brief introductory talk about my injuries and problems. As I was answering questions like, "Do you ever forget to turn off your stove?" I looked into the audience and saw a pair of large brown eyes and a perfectly comforting smile. I directed my subsequent answers to this friendly face, which continued to smile through the duration of the speech. After class, we naturally gravitated toward one another.

"I'm Amanda," she said, "and I'm planning to study nursing or medicine. I'd like to know more about your experiences." From that day on I had my own personal angel at Salem College. She was one of the first college peers who accepted me as myself, ignored my halting speech, laughed at my sometimes witless jokes, and hugged me whenever I had a bad day. I was enough for Amanda, and we remain close friends today.

It was through Amanda and her personal tragedies that I learned to abandon my exalted view of myself—the view that I had more problems than anyone else. Until Amanda, I was intolerant of those with, for instance, anorexia, which I perceived to be a self-inflicted tragedy. She taught me perspective, tolerance, and most of all, the importance of striving for seemingly impossible dreams.

To back up a bit, Amanda's mother died when Amanda was in high school. Her mother was a woman who dreamed of college for her child, but had few financial resources. Amanda was determined to fulfill her late mother's dream.

So she appeared at Salem on a full scholarship after attending a community college for her first two college years. Her family's support was not the monetary kind, and she always had several jobs. Amanda often worked as a Certified Nursing Assistant (CNA) in the local ER at night, and attended classes during the day. She modeled on weekends, and basically did anything legal she could do to pay for the gas in her wreck of a car.

She was never bitter as I often was. She laughed all the time, and made me laugh with her. Amanda helped me relax when faced with some collegiate nuance or the occasional poor mark on an assignment or quiz. I wished I could feel similarly towards the rest of the girls at Salem.

With Amanda I became brave enough to attend classes at Wake Forest University (our schools had reciprocity). I was still afraid to risk the lives of passengers, so she would cart me along with the windows down in her car. We sang Limp Bizkit songs at the top of our lungs through the streets of Winston-Salem. I dared to sing... and my voice wasn't so awful when traveling at high speeds.

Perhaps even more meaningful than anything else, I had become close friends with Amanda on my own. My mother hadn't intervened by inviting her over for a home-cooked meal, and my father hadn't needed to drive me anywhere to visit her. I had cultivated this friendship on my own, and because of that mere fact, it was all the more meaningful. By the time I entered a Wake Forest classroom filled with strangers, I no longer cared if my answers were slightly off center, or if I did badly on a quiz for a teacher who didn't know my background. I remember taking Religion with Amanda. I merely audited that Wake Forest class, which she took for credit. I was still too afraid to fail a class beyond Salem walls. Yet being with my new friend was more than enough excitement for me.

One other new experience I recall was actually more pathetic than exciting.

"I have found us a job," Amanda exclaimed happily, "that pays us each $100 this Saturday! All we have to do is let hairstylists cut our hair at their weekend convention."

"Sure," I said. After all, who wouldn't take a free haircut and $100? I was happy to be a hair model... until we were "blotched!" In the late '90s, hair blotching was a very brief (thank heavens) fad that entailed placing hair dye on the stylist's flat hand, and placing the dye on the back of someone's head. Amanda and I came home with the money and terrible haircuts—and large portions of our hair dyed in different neon colors. The left side of my head was blonde, the back was brown, and the other side was a deep burgundy. The ends and the hair on top of my head were black instead of highlighted blonde. All Amanda did was cry. For once in her life, she was without words. In the end it cost more than $200 to undo the damage. But, hey, we had fun. She was daring, and I wasn't. Slowly she helped me find my inner child again.

At night, on her few evenings free, Amanda and I would sneak into the basement of our dorm and talk. Red wine would occasionally intervene, as we discussed the pros and cons of our love lives. We'd never liked each other's boyfriends, and it turned out we were both right in our analyses. The men just didn't measure up in the end. We both wanted so much for each other, but no one was ever good enough.

I've focused on the social difficulties of college, neglecting the academic. Adolescents need social approval, peer love. I wanted to be normal and fit into a normal peer group, have normal fun, and date a normal guy who wouldn't suffer from watching my TBI-related handicaps. Looking back, I now know that the "academics" were the hardest obstacles; yet as I overcame each new crisis, my self-esteem improved. What did I want from classes then? Knowledge?

"I want A's," I told my parents. "They make me know I'm still smart. They make my friends know I'm smart and not someone who hasn't fully recovered yet." As friends in high school had once defined me, "old Kelly" was reappearing and she wanted to come back. Even though new acquaintances weren't aware of my character traits before the accident, I knew. I had been much more confident before I was broken.

So I went after elusive A's at all costs, tormenting teachers until they gave me extra credit assignments and allowed me to rewrite each paper. I went after A's one course at a time, and with each one, my self-image grew whole again. But the process wasn't easy for anyone.

Once I finally began to receive modifications, especially note-takers and extended time, I could focus well on class lectures. I listened. I stayed after classes to ask questions. If I forgot what I learned in history class, I could always go back and read Xeroxed notes. I didn't tape record lectures because I didn't have time to listen to them. I didn't have stable hands to take notes from a tape. One class at a time, one teacher at a time, I made sure the professors knew me. I took them my medical data, sat in the front row, and made eye contact with each one. I signed up for more advanced courses, and dropped the ones I couldn't handle. This whole process was exhausting, but nothing in me would allow time for extended breaks.

In 1996 I didn't expect college teachers to know about TBI because few did. In high school teachers were uninformed and untrained to help me, but most Salem teachers figured me out somehow. Salem's faculty included many compassionate professors who clearly understood disability issues. My history teacher was amazing.

"What kind of test is best for you? Short answer? Essay? Just tell me what you need, and I will test you accordingly," he said. There were also instructors who made me feel like they shouldn't have to bother with modifications for one student only, but even they eventually understood my perspective.

One course which was mandatory for graduation was taught by a foreign professor, and his accent was so thick I could barely understand him. I was already having a hard enough time responding to most collegiate instructors with their heavily analytical questions, so throwing an accent into the mix didn't help. After the first class I remember running to my advisor's office, and luckily she was there. I burst into her door, forgetting to knock, and began telling her. Just then I realized she was meeting with an advisee's parents.

"I am *so sorry* for my intrusion," I said as I quickly closed the door.

Three minutes later, Ms. Tilley came out and sat down next to me on a bench in the hall. She told the parents that my interruption must be an emergency because such behavior simply was not tolerated at Salem.

"Kelly, why would you enter my private office without as much as a knock?" she almost yelled.

I must have appeared utterly forlorn to her at that moment, and she quickly apologized and gave me a hug. I told her about the difficulty I had with my professor's accent and she shocked me with a smile. Apparently other students had similar concerns about the professor.

Ms. Tilley assured me the teacher usually provided clear and coherent outlines of every class he gave, and she would make sure he did this for me at future sessions. I began to feel better, but my heart rate remained high for the rest of the day.

In my freshman English class I made lots of mistakes, like when we studied Haiku, a rhyme of three lines based on 5 syllables, then 7, then a final 5. I liked my homework poems, but I used a pattern of 3-5-3. Woops! But I liked my eleven-syllable pattern. I decided to make a new kind of poem and call them *oncets* (for the number eleven *once* in Spanish). These are my best ones:

Albatross
Fly higher. Escape
My arrow.

Memories
Add longevity
To moments.

I can't seem to write genuine haiku.

One good move I made was to repeat my first year of foreign language, Spanish I. I had taken it in junior high, and then repeated it in high school. Salem permitted this one more time, so I again took Spanish I. While the material was similar each time, Spanish on the collegiate level was much more difficult. I did, however, pass the class for the third time, my third "A."

Perhaps possessing a little too much confidence in my Spanish speaking ability, I decided to try Conversational Spanish. Not only were students asked to memorize numerous vocabulary words, but many were irregular verbs. When I learned my mid-term and semester exams would ask me to use hundreds of new verbs in conversational form, conjugating tenses appropriately, I decided to drop the course. I knew this would be an impossible feat for my memory, but I'm grateful for the Spanish professor who offered to assist me in any way possible.

"Te puedo dar un banco de palabra, si a usted le gustaria?" Or, "I can give you a word bank if you would like it?" It took me a minute to mentally translate and then process what I was being told.

"Gracias." I stammered "Pero estoy bien." Thanks, I had told her, but I'm fine. I could see myself memorizing the required data after many hours of repetition, but ultimately chose to replace Conversational Spanish with a course in creative writing, which I excelled in. Comprehensive exams, I'd learned, were not best for students with TBI.

In the creative writing course I wasn't required to memorize anything. I simply learned a more specific method to write in. I would decide the content of a story and the characters to use. I then chose a point of view and began to write short fiction.

Through writing, I discovered my imagination had been subdued until I began composing creatively. My Communication classes also involved a lot of writing, with no time limitations. My writing skills improved and I made more A's easily. However, after turning in each paper or test, I still became paralyzed with fear. Would I fail? What would happen if I failed?

I recall one particular "Com" test which almost destroyed me. It was long, and my hand shook so hard that the pencil nearly fell onto the floor. I absolutely could not sleep that night, so I called and e-mailed my professor. He didn't answer. I went to his office—not there! So I drove around Salem Square the next day until I spotted him parking his car. He looked up and saw my worried face.

"You got an A, Kelly... as always!" Chip Cox yelled across the street. And I could breathe again. I was still smart. And so the process continued. I studied. I typed. I dictated assignments to my mother, my scribe, when pains shot up my arms. I took difficult classes in summer school. In those, I labored for B's. Somehow I failed no college class, but I did have to be clever and self-advocate.

12 On My Own

"Never be afraid to try something new. Remember, amateurs built the ark; professionals built the *Titanic*."
– Unknown

I became brave enough to attend summer classes at UNC-Chapel Hill, living with high school friend Nicole Price. The summer session went well; I made a B with no modifications—and a change of academic environment was very refreshing. I could walk to all classes. One night I made chocolate chip cookies for the crew of *Patch Adams* filming nearby, and an appreciative cameraman gave me a costuming job. I got to know the crew and cast (including Robin Williams) as real people. My life was improving, but I attributed my newfound confidence to living in a new city where no one knew my disability level. Surely, my TBI symptoms could improve if I changed where I lived.

The next two summers, I made sure I was elsewhere. One year I interned with Community Living of Wilmington, and co-produced a Mary Chapin Carpenter Concert. My boss lent me her cell phone, and I called her each time I got lost in the city. With the Atlantic Ocean limiting the possibilities, I managed my directional issues much better. Another summer I traveled to Merida, Mexico, with a group from Peace College, Raleigh, NC. Simply writing a journal of my experiences there gave me course credit at Salem in several subjects. Despite dengue fever, minor floods, and life without air-conditioning, I realized how happy I was in a foreign atmosphere. Jenny Port, a newfound friend, helped me negotiate the strange streets of a Mexican city. My parents made sure I was supervised by a friend in the Spanish department of Peace, but I felt blissfully, briefly unaware of watchful eyes taking care of me.

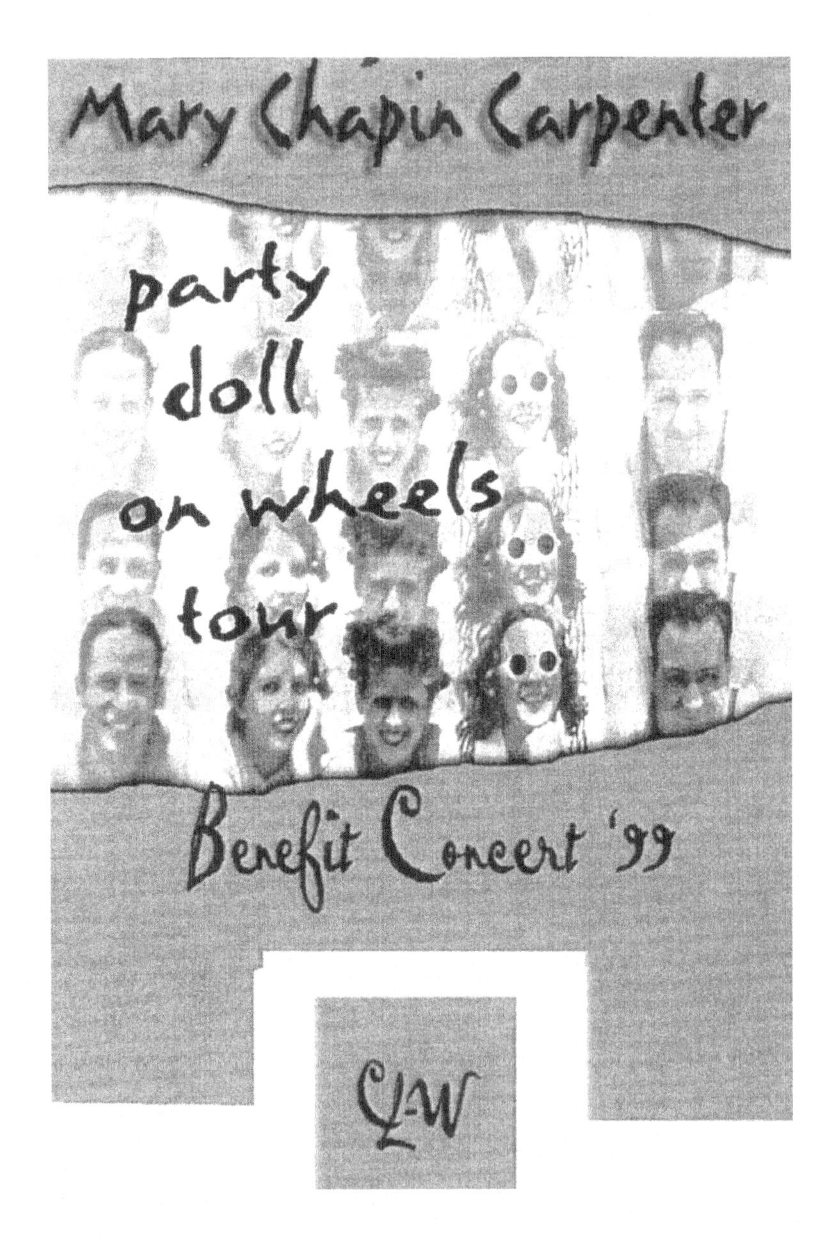

Mary Chapin Carpenter poster, Community Living of Wilmington, NC

However, this Mexican trip, plus two class trips to Europe, did increase my personal anger with a life of limitations. I wanted to fly far away and leave all TBI issues behind me. But it doesn't work that way, as disabilities tend to follow you wherever you hide.

One January during college, I interned for a local television station. I basically observed reporters and was allowed to practice running the station's cameras. While working late nights there, I met and flirted with an unusually attractive guy and proceeded to break up with Lee. The really cute guy was not my only reason. I've included an excerpt from my mother's journal about this event:

> Well, I knew this day was coming. I've dreaded this January since October, but I never realized how painful and difficult it would be. Months ago, Kelly brought me a liability release form from Salem College, asking parental permission for her to intern with a local television station during her January Term (60 hour class compacted into one month, for her major). She planned to get rides or drive herself while still afraid of the Interstate (another of her self-imposed tests, perhaps necessary). After days of loud arguing she agreed to abide by whatever rules her father and I set, if she could accept the job. I signed, thinking of ice storms and certain arguments to follow. I knew I was committing Bobby to a long, tedious practicing period on the roadways between Salem and the TV station out on I-40 East. Driving had been his one main area of responsibility. He did need an arm twist as they hadn't practiced new routes in the last year.
>
> The week before Christmas, Kelly hugged me tight in one of our late-night talks. She said that she knew she would be safe because I believed that she could do it. Pressure? I rarely knew what was safe or what wasn't.
>
> Soon Bobby and Kelly began practicing back routes along country roads to the station, then the Interstate route, which was far shorter. By January 1st, Kelly thought she probably knew the way. She began the internship driving on lengthy back roads, working the 9 a.m. to 5 p.m. shift. She was so proud of herself! Then, unexpectedly, she moved her shift to 11 a.m. to 7 p.m. There were probably more cute guys working in the evenings. We didn't scream because on this shift she would avoid rush hour traffic. At this point, she graduated from back roads to the quick few miles on the Interstate. Against enor-

mous protest, Bobby followed her home a few nights, although staying up so late was hard for him. His job required early hours. Finally, we let her drive alone. Two nights later, she turned the wrong way and got lost somewhere in Kernersville, NC. Bobby returned to his 'following,' for he was terrified she would enter the Interstate on an approach ramp. Sometimes she didn't know he was there. He hid his car behind a billboard and tailed her like a plainclothes policeman.

Then came what I call "the *Titanic* influence." She had seen the famous Leonardo DiCaprio movie, and one young cameraman at the television station was a ringer for the actor. Naturally he was flirting hard with Kelly, who always looked like she hadn't a disability in the world. She began to alter her schedule more and more, working until midnight at the station, and once until 1:30 a.m. Kelly was declaring her independence from family and from Lee and others in her support network. She wanted the freedom to make her own decisions, even if she wrecked her car at midnight. "I can't be a part of this family anymore," she declared. Thus Bobby and I had to "let go" and allow Kelly to find her own social and physical parameters. We stayed at home, waiting for the phone to ring again. I began having panic attacks. Even lying on my den floor with arms outstretched, the world would spin and spin until I would finally fall asleep. The *Titanic* would sink, but maybe my child would find a place on a lifeboat.

In brief, Kelly broke off her three-year relationship with Lee. Her reasons were strangely sound, if adolescent. "I can't live my whole life being Lee's shadow," Kelly exclaimed. "I want to see if I can fit into the world on my own. Lee can't spend his life simply taking me where I need to go, and doing whatever I ask. He's in college now and isn't making friends because he's always with me. I have to stand alone, and he has to have the chance at a normal life. The only gift I can give him is normalcy."

I have tried to tell her that there is no such thing as a normal life, but clearly she must find that out for herself.

Kelly also got lost a few more times. She has a terrible tendency to make right turns, ending up where she started. When she's home, all conversations end up in arguments. I'm very tired. I listen and listen to her pleas for fewer rules.

> Sometimes I make a point and she actually hears me. Bob is also having stress symptoms, and has begun to meet privately with Dr. Mattox.
>
> It seems that Bobby and I, and also Lee, represent barriers to Kelly—not the safety nets we once were. We are letting go as fast as we can. Our goal is the same: her independence. I thought that because Kelly spent months and years in hospitals and rehabilitation centers, we got to skip the ups and downs of adolescence! But she is now back to her old fifteen-year-old self. Only this time she's inside the body of a nineteen-year-old. I know my daughter is wiser than before. She's gotten better by denying obstacles and persevering, but now I must help her to admit she is not, and never will be, as free as her college comrades. Acceptance of limitations, and some sound judgment of men, will be goals for the next year.
>
> Kelly was a debutante this year! She showed the world how lovely she is once again. Her "hidden illness" didn't show, but I am having nightmares. I am remembering a phone call to Lee when Kelly's beloved golden retriever died. She was in an exam, so we chose not to tell her. Lee and his brother Jon dug a grave for Dustey, spending hours making the corners perfect. Lee placed Dustey's nose facing Kelly's bedroom window so he could watch over her forever. Kelly is too immersed in her recovery to recognize what love really is. Earlier today I accepted Kelly's resignation from the family. I wonder how long it will last.

Well, it lasted three days. I came home and cried myself sick and threw up a lot. My tears disappeared in 1992 and haven't come back yet. My mother said I was self-sabotaging by releasing Lee.

"He sees you as perfect, you see something damaged," my mother said. I remember her exact words. Every time I was tempted to call Lee and beg forgiveness, I thought of the damage I might do to his future, and didn't call. I clung to Amanda, but I needed more.

I needed a lot of guardian angels in college, and yes, Amanda was definitely one… she remains my best friend today. The others were the people who told me the truth, which was not always what I wanted to hear. Relationships were so hard for me because I felt I always let people down. Dates were almost impossible yet I wanted to date and do the "normal college" things. I became a master of pretense, ever striving to prove my normalcy, trying to prove I was not in any way inferior. I would go to bars or frat parties dressed in my most stylish clothes (often chosen by my suitemates because I easily forgot which clothes went with which shoes, or even which clothes I owned. If I couldn't see clothing in the front of the closet, I rarely dug to the back to look for a matching outfit). I flirted easily, because at parties no one cares about anything but superficial looks and laughter. Later, if a guy asked me out, I had to explain that I couldn't drive a car on highways, and I couldn't drink very much. By the time my diatribe was over, the guy had either left or was bored out of his mind. Sometimes my relationships lasted for several dates, but only until the boys figured out that casual sex was not one of the plans for the evening.

Amanda, however, encouraged me to get out and look for someone worthy. I did flirt easily, but often preferred being "point man" for girlfriends. Why? I'll tell you about my date with Fred, an intern at Forsyth Hospital.

"Let's go to the opera," he said. "Do you like *La Traviata*?"

"Sure," I replied. And I went to my first opera.

"You on the pill?" he asked at intermission

"Nope," I responded. I couldn't think of another word to say all evening. Frederick actually called me again, but I made excuses not to go out with him. He terrified me despite my real and present interest in medicine. This man was eight years older than I, sophisticated, sexy, and smart. And I wasn't ready to cope. I'm more of a *U2* girl.

Instead of dating constantly, I turned to girlfriends—yes, finally I had those by my third college year. Some, like me, were disabled. "Gardner" was a beautiful opera major and was deaf in one ear. The girls on my hall junior year were all wonderful, kind human beings. With Kristy and others, I went on my first real "Spring Break" to abandon the studious life and meet people who didn't care about issues like TBI. The Carnival Cruise line was offering a special package, so off we went to discover St. Lucia and other beautiful islands. I met a New Yorker named Matt who had just finished his MBA. And I learned to gamble. My card sense and my affinity for numbers were intact, and at first Matt and I attempted blackjack. We won more than we lost and moved to the roulette wheel in the corner. With a few hundred dollars in his pocket, Matt said, "Kelly, where do we put the money?" For some reason, I thought about my dark experience on 9/17/92, and said, "Put all of it on Black 17!"

The wheel kept spinning and stopped where I knew it would. Cheers around the room—Black 17 won hundreds for us that night.

What were the odds? About as great as going out for a sandwich and having a TBI? Then the next morning our group disembarked in St. Thomas. I'd told Matt I wasn't scared of much other than spiders and mimes (Tyler and I despised them), but I didn't want him to leave me lost on a foreign street. Suddenly we saw a black and white fellow appear in full costume—a mime! He crawled along the wooden dock, met my horrified stare, then leapt up, grabbed me and kissed me hard. I spat and ran away. What were the odds of that?

I pondered "odds" often after that cruise. I thought about all my "second birthday parties," when each year my parents would say, "You were nineteen on September 12th, and four on the 17th!" They celebrated my second life as a gift, and always remembered it. Each time my parents would light candles on a second cake, I realized, "What were the odds of my having a mother trained in special education?" Finally I had something new to believe in—the odds. I probably won't win twice on Black 17, or have another TBI. I'd reject another mother. The odds spoke to me—I'd probably find a life worth living if I looked long enough. And someone to love the imperfect me. I felt strangely calm after that spring break. My friends understood my issues, having problems of their own... which I now recognized. I wasn't alone anymore. In fact, I was facing what all college graduates face—the inevitable approach of adulthood and work!

13 Graduation and Employment

"We are all phenomenal women!"
–Aisha Dew, Salem Class of 2000

In 2000 I graduated from college cum laude with departmental honors in Communication, and Oprah Winfrey was our graduation speaker. Oprah was very close to the incomparable Dr. Maya Angelou, who lived and taught at Wake Forest University in Winston-Salem, and Maya's niece Rosa, or "the Rose" Johnson was in my class at Salem. Rosa and others in my class had bombarded Oprah with phone calls, e-mails, gifts, and pleading words to convince her to come and address us, and she finally agreed.

"You're relentless," she said. "You don't know how to take no for an answer. You're my kind of women." We were thrilled beyond words. Oprah's own words to us were sometimes very personal, addressed to specific individuals who had written to her the past year. I remember how affected I was by her confessions and perspectives when she talked about empowerment.

"Real power," she said, "is when you are doing exactly what you are supposed to be doing, the best it can be done. Authentic power. There's a surge; there's a kind of energy field that says, 'I'm in my groove,' and nobody has to tell you 'You go, girl,' because you know you're already gone."

Well, I thought about her speech for a long time. I realized that while I rarely knew if my actions were wrong or right, I did feel a sort of "wind at my back" when I was on the right path. Because of Oprah, I try to tap into this feeling when I have big decisions to make. And I try to follow her advice—she said if a young black woman with frizzy hair falling out could make it in the world, then so could each of us, no

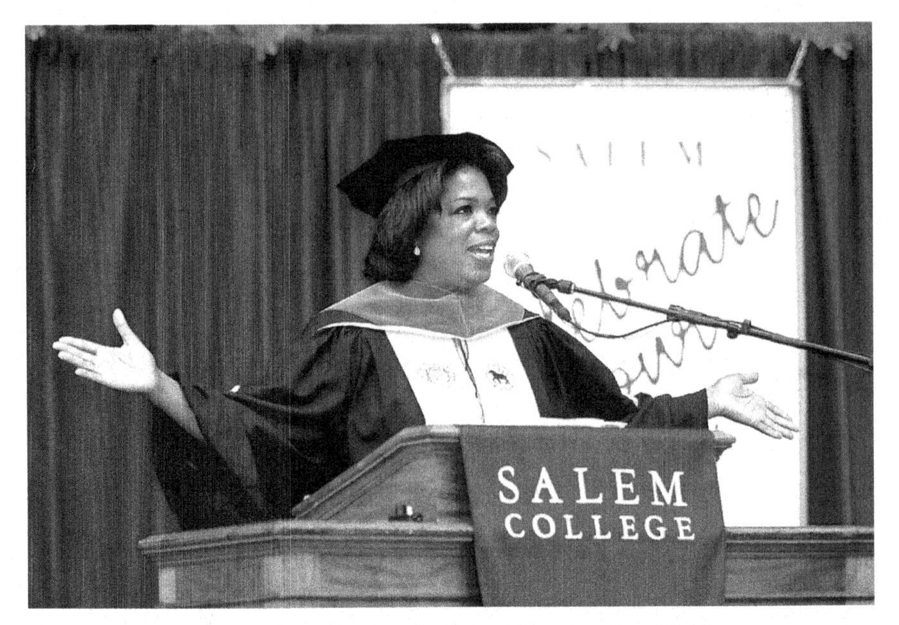

Oprah Winfrey, Salem College graduation 2000

matter what the obstacles. She also told us what she learned from Maya Angelou—not to worry so much about what others think.

"You give yourself the authority to be what you were meant to be. You don't even need a *man*!" Oprah said and the whole graduating class applauded. "You are the author of your own life." Okay, so TBI was my obstacle, and I couldn't let it stop me from living a life with purpose and joy.

During graduation weekend, I made a great error. I refused a position in the admissions office of Salem College. Guaranteed employment? I didn't care. I wanted to leave the city of my pain. What did I know about health benefits in 2000? The light hadn't dawned—I needed to support myself in a time of no Obamacare. My parents couldn't keep me on their insurance policy. I had to go to work, and had no idea what to do.

I looked arduously for employment outside of Winston-Salem, but it proved to be a much harder task than I thought. The highways out of town were intimidating, and no job with health benefits cried out for a graduate recovering from severe traumatic brain injury. Once I spun out on a major highway and had to call a friend to escort me home from the grassy median. Thankfully, no one was hurt. If circumstances had been fractionally different, the results could have been disastrous. Realizing this, I never again drove on highways.

Turning my focus back to my hometown, I sought out an employment attorney. He told me what I did and didn't need to tell prospective employers about TBI. I went back to WFU/BMC to the Neuropsychology Department and attended mock interviews to help assess my skills. As recommended, I applied for jobs with non-profit organizations. Hopefully, they could use my writing and interpersonal skills.

I eventually accepted a position with the American Red Cross (ARC) in Winston-Salem. I was their Volunteer Shift Coordinator, and was paid to ensure ample staffing at every blood drive at varying locations, as well as at the permanent facility. The hours at the Red Cross were long. Blood drives could be held 361 days a year. Thus with funds from an "insurance-based trust", I bought a small condominium less than a mile from work, and even on Sunday mornings was passing out Krispy Kreme doughnuts to donors who helped save lives via donated blood.

My job description included finding two adults to be present during each blood drive, and this quota was reasonably difficult. The records of the local Red Cross were on worn index cards, so with my technology skills, I computerized their databank of volunteers (one very long weekend). Many of my friends and my parents' friends gave me volunteer hours that year, and yes, they were part of my personal flight of angels. They gave me time, which my grandfather had told me "is the only true gift."

Surely anyone's first full-time position is frightening, but I was terrified that my short-term memory issues would hinder my ability to find volunteers for the ARC.

Somehow, in the rushed atmosphere of donations, I forgot to be overwhelmed. I analyzed the volunteer shortage as I analyzed college research. Who would be available besides those close to me? Students needing community service hours, retirees, Mormon missionaries? I began to fill my shifts.

Then I faced another work-related challenge. I had to fully staff each blood drive held throughout Winston-Salem, in public schools, colleges, and local businesses. For most people, this would be a non-issue, but I had to find these places without using major, heavily traversed roads. I didn't have access to GPS (Global Positioning System) back then. After a few months had passed, I felt slightly more confident with the locales, and probably learned new routes, which I continue using today.

At the time I often called friends and family. "Where is Old Lexington Road? Which way should I turn on Robinhood Road to get home from Tobaccoville?" By then I had a cell phone, which made my life much simpler!

On the rare occasions I forgot to fully staff a blood drive, my mother would graciously take the blame. "Tell them Carolyn is coming. Tell them I'm kind of ditzy, but I'm on my way now!" she would say. After three months, I didn't forget anymore. I learned to be quite responsible, and began to realize my TBI diagnosis had hidden benefits. It turned out that friends were more than willing to volunteer and give blood. They helped me to forge ahead in my first real occupation.

I recall at several high school blood drives, students asked, "Can I give blood if I have an STD or if I might be HIV positive?"

"I would go ahead and give," I suggested. "The Red Cross will screen your blood before sending it to any of the hospitals. The results will be mailed to your home or to any address you provide."

Some kids traded addresses and had their free AIDs test sent to a home other than their own. I hope some lives were saved this way.

Once I organized a blood drive with the Kappa Kappa Gammas of Wake Forest University, where I had previously delivered a TBI awareness speech. These girls planned a blood drive in a campus cafeteria. They staffed it well, but forgot to advertise. Few students showed up to donate blood, and for the first time in years, I forgot I had a handicap. I ran to the center of the cafeteria and jumped up onto a table.

"Please come and donate blood," I called out to the crowd. "If your friends are in accidents, they may need your help. One pint of blood can save up to three lives!"

And students came in large numbers. We ended up having an excellent drive. All I had to do was be outgoing (as people tell me the "old Kelly" would have been).

Gaining confidence in this position, I began to scout graduate programs in various fields. I'd promised to stay for one year at the ARC, but a catastrophic event kept me there longer. It was 9/11. In the midst of a blood drive on the top floor of a high-rise, I watched the towers fall on an enormous wide screen TV. My father was in New York City on business when the Twin Towers were tumbling.

President Bush announced on TV: "If you want to help, go to your local Red Cross and give blood!" This was a huge error. Most Red

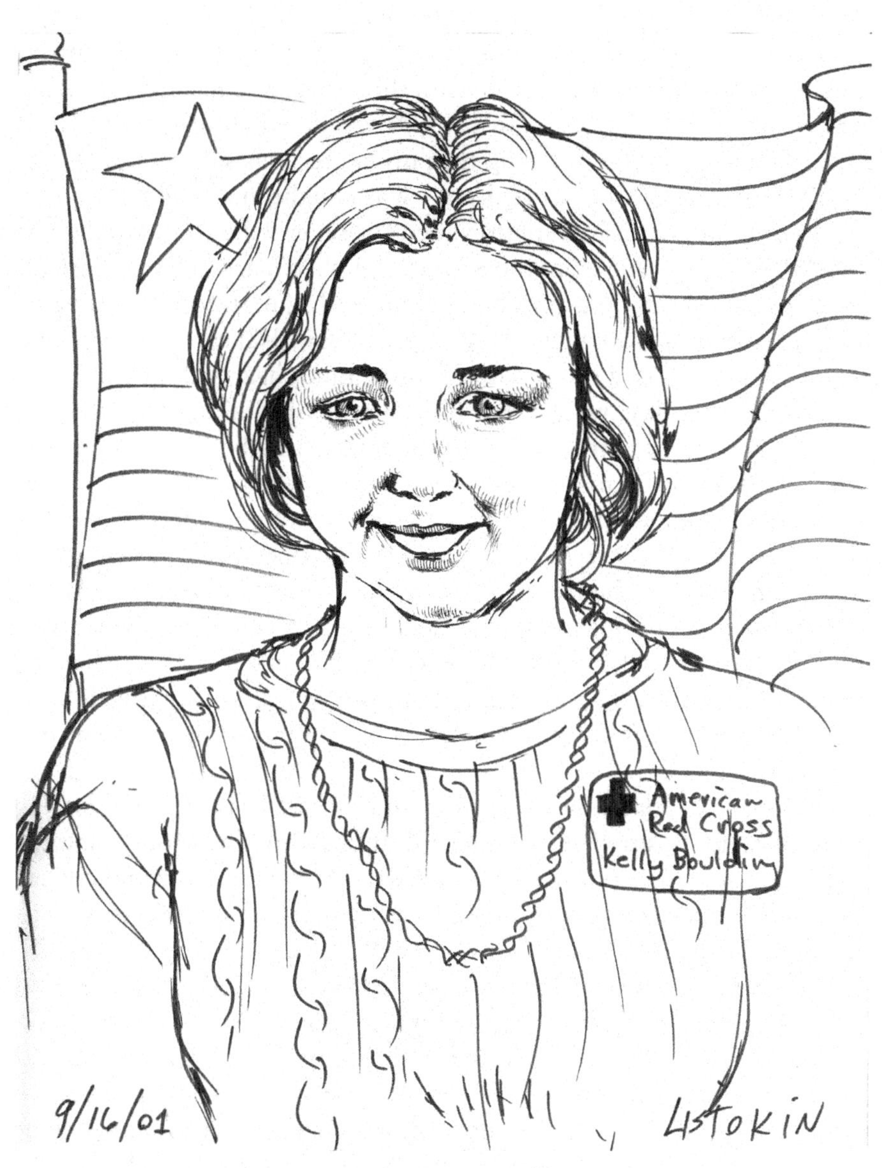

Kelly five days after 9/11 at ARC (Winston-Salem)

Cross offices don't have the capacity to refrigerate gallons upon gallons of blood for long periods. Initially, neither the Red Cross nor the public thought of this, but after a short time, the realization began to dawn. Meanwhile in Winston-Salem, thousands of concerned students and citizens parked along Coliseum Drive and tried to storm the Red Cross offices. After confirming that my father was safely on a bridge on the outskirts of NYC, I realized I was caught in a mob.

A communal atmosphere prevailed for several days (and nights) at the ARC, like a scene from the Sixties.... A sketch artist drew charcoal pictures of donors, and musicians sang with guitar accompaniment. College students were picnicking on our lawn. What were we, at the Red Cross, supposed to do with all these kind, heartsick people?

For the first day, we worked hour after hour, taking blood donations. Then word came, the sad word, that this blood wouldn't be needed after all; too many were dead in the aftermath of 9/11. We set up more telephones and worked the crowds, taking appointments for future donations. We sent blood to states that needed it. It was chaos and confusion, yet the feeling of community prevailed at the ARC.

This was a turning point moment in my adult life. I was alive, period. How could I complain about a bad memory and shaking hands? I may have had a traumatic brain injury, but my disabilities hadn't mattered in this crisis. In fact, I was humbled by my own self-preoccupation.

After a reasonable grace period, one of the best 9/11 volunteers took over my position as volunteer shift coordinator. Months later, I began a new career pursuit, one that would lead me to special education and writing. I missed my Red Cross associates, but was joyous to have weekends off at last.

Occasionally, when I had a few spare hours, I dated a friend named Jim who said, "I hate to see you alone so much." And so I adopted a dog, a mutt who had been abused. She's a tiny brown fuzzball named Macy who likes to catch Frisbees and who suffers from obsessive compulsive disorder (OCD). Those big brown eyes of hers can see right into your heart. I finally had a warm body to share my bed at night, and a soft shoulder to cry on. My Macy taught me more about love than anyone had in a long time.

Have you ever read any novels by Dean Koontz? There usually is at least one heroic dog functioning as the protagonist (as in the novels *Watchers* and *Breathless*). Well, sometimes I was the antagonist of my own life story, ever trying to be more or less than I was and am. I hated

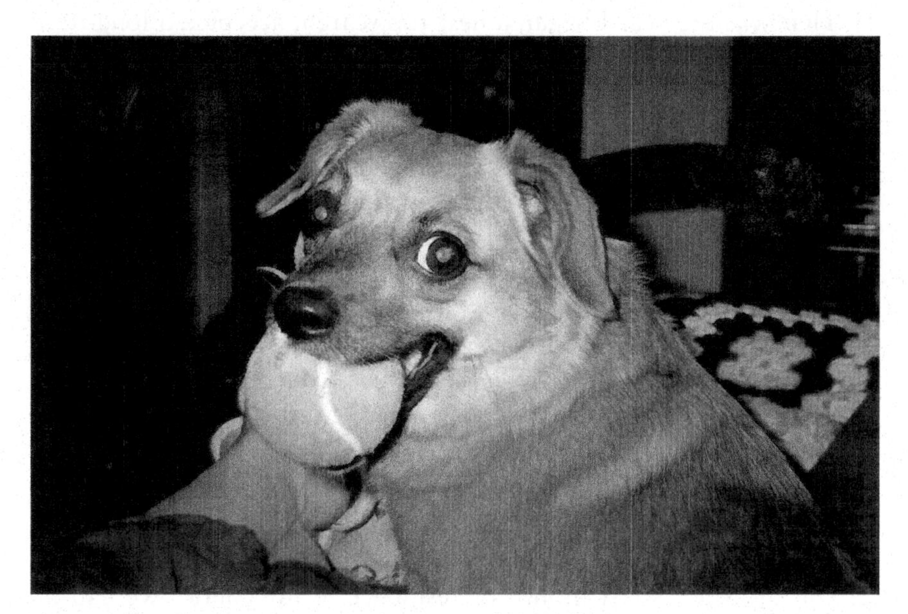

Macy with her Ball-Ball

my own imperfections, and still felt that any decent man deserved more than I could possibly offer. I tended to engage in relationships with needful men who could accept my flaws because I willingly embraced theirs. Macy, however, did not accept less than she wanted. She taught me to aim for the moon, even if I fell in the stars.

About that time, my beautiful sister Tyler became engaged. I was Maid of Honor at her wedding and met one of her husband's groomsmen, Evan. He came to visit me several weeks later. He was completing his final college semester online, and began looking for part-time work in Winston-Salem. I allowed him to abandon his own apartment search to stay in my condo for weeks. I helped him study. No one could convince me that this man was not my future... except Macy.

One night Evan was lying on the bed, and my gentle mutt hopped up on the coverlet I'd saved to purchase. Macy never had accidents in the condo, never nipped or destroyed property. She was pure love and joy.

I watched as Macy sniffed quietly at Evan's foot and nosed his clothing. Macy then raised her leg and peed on him. She gazed up at me with a look that said: "Not the right one!"

That was the year I began a new job search, accepted a long-term substituting position, and applied for graduate school in special education. Evan left. I had my work, a great dog, and a new challenge in graduate school.

To pay my mortgage I took a job at Smiley-Fitness by Design, a fitness center across from my condo, and for the first time since 1992 became physically strong again. I made a variety of new friends of all ages, and took graduate classes full-time. My parents stopped by often to walk Macy, and eventually 'stole' her away from me. They fell in love with her, too, and perhaps the hardest thing I've done is to let her stay with them permanently. She still gives her "mamma" kisses, and I see her every day. I waited until marriage and a fenced-in yard to rescue mutts again. Over time I realized I had given my father something he'd lost in '92—laughter in the house! For no special reason, I'd taught Macy commands backwards. She eats "creamice" and "cornpop," and runs on the "walkside" chasing "munkchips."

During Macy's last month of residence in my condo, we had an unusual night that was typical of my more "bi-polar" moments. At midnight Macy jumped on my bed in her vulture position—two paws on my chest and a nose between my eyes. This meant "bathroom break," but was far later than our usual trip to the "doo doo place" behind the building. But she wouldn't relent despite my head buried under the pillows. I struggled up, grabbed her leash, and went outside in my nightclothes.

The stars were very bright outside, and I watched as the Diamondback Bar and Grill across the street shut down its lights. Macy and I wandered around, taking care of her business. I felt peaceful. Responsible. Taking good care of Macy meant I'd be a capable mother someday, one who wouldn't forget to change a diaper, or remember doctors' appointments. I reached for my doorknob. Woops, I hadn't left it cracked. The key I usually carried in my jeans pocket was inside with my blue jeans.

I had a spare key hidden in my car. Naturally, this too was locked, the keys inside my purse in the condo. Soon I was banging on my next-door neighbor's door, and he reluctantly let me in to call and wake my parents. They quickly came and let me inside, but I felt terribly low. I'm sure this event doesn't sound unusual to anyone who ever locked themselves out.

But I did it again the following night. Going outside to get better reception on my cell phone, I unconsciously closed my back door, and it got locked with Macy still inside. Again I called my parents because, fortunately, my cell was in my hand.

"It's no big deal," said my father at 11 p.m. "But you need to hide a key!"

Well, I had hidden keys, but my memory strategies were still not succeeding. My mental computer was busy recalling the details of work, and deleting the "trivia" of independent living. I asked myself, "What did you do before, when you couldn't solve a problem?" My inner self spoke: "You asked a friend for help."

I called my cousin Marc from work the next day because he lived in a nearby condo, and he was smart and sympathetic. He knew I concentrated hard on the requirements of new courses, to the detriment of details at home. A house key was like an ignored "pop-up window" in a brain filled with important downloads.

"Get another extra key," Marc said, "and put it in one of those 'hiding rocks' you see on TV. But put the hiding rock under my porch stoop, not yours. That way, if someone finds it, they won't break into your house."

Such an obvious solution, and I hated myself for not thinking of it first. And then I thought, "I did a good thing by consulting a smart person." I wasn't a total imbecile. Ironically, after planting the hidden rock at Marc's, I never locked myself out again. Macy wasn't locked in or out alone again.

14 The Master's Degree: Prognosis and Possibilities

"The principal goal of education is to create men who are capable of doing new things, not simply of repeating what other generations have done."

- Jean Piaget

Most of the classes in Salem College's Graduate School were held during evening hours, and the professors were very tolerant of students with disabilities. I assumed all instructors teaching us of the Individuals with Disabilities Education Act (IDEA), and how to effectively write an Individualized Education Plan (IEP), would be willing to modify their own tests for a student with TBI. But that wasn't the case.

In one of my reading courses, my instructor refused to give me extended time to write discussion questions for his final exam... and there I was with a bilateral hand impairment—documented. While I hadn't planned for any such confrontation on the graduate level in an education course, I'd learned to prepare for the unexpected. I made an appointment with the head of the Master of Arts in Teaching program in Education to discuss my instructor's astonishing neglect of my needs.

After several days of debating for and against my need for modifications ("But you're in grad school now!" said the professor), I was granted word banks of pertinent terms for essay writing, and extended time to complete the exam. My professor did, however, expect me to remain within the graduate school building while taking the exam.

Teachers in the past had allowed me to take tests home to complete in a more relaxed setting. This change of environment would calm my anxieties so that I could write more easily and with much more confidence. I naturally had signed several copies of Salem's honor code before completing tests at home, but my professor didn't yield. He agreed to stay in the building until I completed his essay questions manually.

The evening of my exam finally arrived and I'd taken off work that day to study. When I received the test, I sought a remote corner of the building so as not to be disturbed. I began filling in the short answers, and thinking through each of my discussion questions. I opened my laptop, made outlines for each and began to write. With my hand impairment, my typing speed was still approximately 18 words per minute. When my trembling became too severe, I took small breaks to stretch out my fingers. At three in the morning, I printed out my essays and went to my professor's office to turn them in. He appeared a bit disheveled, in desperate need of rest, and he gladly accepted my completed exam.

I made a B on the exam and a B+ in the course. I have since heard the secretary of the graduate school say that this professor never again refused to give modifications to students in need of extended time. I guess I had needed to prove my needs were justified that night, but I still wonder why my professor couldn't simply believe what I'd told him. This was a "Special Ed" program.

In the final semester of graduate school, I was required to pass the Praxis II (a standardized test used to evaluate knowledge of students with varying disability levels) in my area of expertise, to obtain my specialized teaching license. Hearing of this test sent me into an immediate panic attack... more testing, more phone calls, more letters, more begging for accommodations and more attempts at crossing the "red tape jungle" with the Praxis II. Following a long talk with my mother, I decided to go for it. I would try my hardest to acquire accommodations for the Praxis II. All I could now do was study, study, study.

"Will you work with me this one last time, and help me pass the Praxis II in my subject area?" I begged. If my mother agreed, she was saying she believed I could pass. She had always been honest with me, and promised in the hospital to remain so. This meant a great deal since most friends still said basically what I wanted to hear.

"Of course," she replied. "We always have so much fun studying together." I inherited her sarcasm.

After researching various testing sites, the closest one was NC Central University (NCCU), in Durham, North Carolina. Durham is about an hour and a half from Winston-Salem, which meant my father would have to drive me to the testing site. After much discussion, we agreed on traveling to Durham the day before the Praxis II, spending the night in a nearby hotel and getting up early the next morning to take the exam.

I had informed the appropriate people at Salem that I would need additional time to complete the matching and discussion questions. This exam was administered on a computer and would be timed by a person working in the building.

The day before the test, my mother and I had been doing what we did best—studying, studying, studying. After my father left work, we went to Durham. We'd enlisted my Aunt LaLa to stay with Macy. Once we were checked into our hotel room, my mother and I went into study-and-review mode. We both purchased soft drinks and took my review materials down to the pool area so we could study outside. Doing something depressing (like overlearning) was always easier for me outside, calmed by nature.

Mother kept repeating numerous fill-in-the-blank questions, giving me several choices for the correct answer. I did well on our review session that evening, which greatly elevated my self-confidence. The following day, I awoke feeling rested, ready to take the exam.

My father, mother, and I crammed into my dad's white Crown Victoria and drove to NCCU. We found the correct building with ease, yet my mother and I went inside only to be told that there was no record of my need for extended time. My heart froze and everything in my head began to jumble—a flood. In Claudia Osborn's book, *Over My Head*, she used "flooding" to describe an overwhelming sensation felt by a person with TBI in which the victim can't recall his or her name much less the answer to a simple question. The elderly African-American man administering the exam noticed my terror, and chuckled. He assured me that even though there was no record of my need for modification, he would give me the time-and-a-half.

"Happens all the time," he said. "I hate to see potential teachers wasted... let me see the documentation you brought with you. I'll explain the computer test now. You'll be fine!"

I looked up at him and beamed a smile of appreciation. Again I could breathe, think. I was reminded once more of the influence people in lower places possess. I learned afterwards that the man had given me as much time as I needed and perhaps moments more. Not only did I pass the Praxis II, I received one of the highest scores in North Carolina for that testing period.

One of my last requirements for graduate school was student teaching for a semester. I was placed in a local middle school and assigned to a class of children categorized as "mild to moderately" disabled. For the layman, this might imply either minor or severe disability. I wondered beforehand if the students' handicaps were greater or less than my own, and hoped I could overcome my memory issues and shaking right hand to truly help this class at all.

I can remember being beside myself with nerves on my first day, but being frightened had never stopped me in the past, so why allow it to now? Also, one of my supervisors, Ms. Vitale, was a favorite professor from grad school. She had promised to keep a close eye on me if I needed assistance.

My first day of student teaching arrived, and it rained. Waking up that morning, I was literally shaking with nerves, anxiety and excitement. I left my condo early enough to compensate for any wrong turns made along the way, later learning that I'd left my front door unlocked and that my mother had discovered this when she came to walk Macy. The entire world seemed soggy.

Shaking, I walked through the ominous double doors of "my" school. My hands were numb and I couldn't breathe well. After the seemingly endless journey to "my" trailer behind the school, I walked into what seemed like another world with a dozen students all doing different things, all in different locations or stations. Some, like Jason, were attentive, focused. Most were quietly sitting at their desks, performing work at their own individual pace. Others seemed rather lost... like me in 1992.

I silently chuckled. I realized very quickly how little I knew about the world of special education. The world I was entering was nothing like textbook predictions, scholarly studies, and filmstrips. This was something quite new to my experience. I took a deep breath and voiced a weak "Hello." And some faces smiled back at me.

Then a thought rose from my subconscious. Were the parents of these students like mine, wanting what teachers call the LRE (least restrictive environment) for their children? Or did they fear the stigma of special categorization? Were they afraid their children wouldn't learn to function independently in life? I would never know their feelings—then. I had many children to study and teach. One would alter my life view forever.

One Monday I was helping students with a social studies assignment, the first full unit of lessons I planned myself. (Sadly, the teachers had to define "unit" for me). The children were asked to color pictures of Roman architecture while they learned about life in ancient Rome. One little boy, Carter, was sitting at his desk, staring at the wall. He had spiky brown hair and long, dirty fingernails. I asked him if he was all right. No response. I asked him again... silence. I placed my hand on his shoulder to ask a third time, and he nearly jumped out of his seat. I emulated his jump and my heart began to race. Yet the lead teacher smiled. I certainly had managed to get his attention.

I asked Carter why he wasn't coloring his pictures of Rome. He looked at me with a questioning expression.

"Aqueducts don't... have any... color," he replied in a whispering, erratic voice. He then grabbed a pencil and began to stab his desk. I told him how smart he was to know that aqueducts were a white, stone color, but then I asked why he was stabbing his desk. He said he was bored and continued stabbing. I asked him to please stop, explaining that other people who worked at the school would have to come into the classroom at night to clean off these markings. He didn't care. I tried to take the pencil and he immediately recoiled back in his seat.

"If you do that again, I'll stab you!" he stated. I must have either had a lot of adrenalin pumping through my system or was just incredibly stupid, but I held out my hand.

"Stab me then... but either way you need to take part in this assignment." He looked up at me with his big brown eyes and slowly put the pencil down.

After a short wait, Carter reached for a crayon and drew a blue aqueduct. I had just experienced my first power struggle with a student. Perhaps I could have handled the situation better by helping him to verbalize his feelings of boredom, but with my expressive difficulties, I didn't see that as a viable option. And I'd been taught that 90% of communication is nonverbal. But as I watched this child calmly coloring, a realization formed.

Carter's handicaps were categorized as "mild to moderate." So what was I? Formerly, my perception of self was that of moderate to severe disability. And I was wrong. I was able to speak, control my behaviors, and learn. And I was through feeling sorry for myself.

After my revelation, after the experience with the potentially lethal pencil, I was on edge the rest of the day. Yet following that encounter, Carter always obeyed my instructions. He became precious to me by the end of my student teaching. All of my experiences at this middle school taught me how truly fortunate I was. And am. I knew I could teach students with TBI, BED (Behavioral and Emotional Disorders) and Autism. The students would be teaching me as I continued to learn and write. I later learned my brightest student was diagnosed as having TBI. Perhaps my career had begun.

Then a small miracle added to my new confidence. This, ironically, occurred on a truly grim day in a graduate class. I was asked to write an original and lengthy comparative analysis on one controversial problem in current American education. Guess what I selected! However, TBI was rejected as a topic for me because not enough studies existed on the topic. I was told there were plenty of medical studies, but no educational studies to compare and contrast. After useless arguing, I was assigned a lengthy diatribe on the advantages vs. disadvantages of peer tutoring.

That night I went home and stayed up most of the night pounding on my computer. "Our teachers are not prepared!" I wrote. For the next few nights I stayed up late writing the paper I had really wanted to write—building off of earlier essays—and took it with me to class. Naturally, I also presented an analysis of peer tutoring (I still wanted my A's). However, some faculty members read my unsolicited views on the dearth of information on students with TBI in American schools. I asked my mother, the teacher, to read it, and she said, "This is publishable." On her advice I sent my text to the *English Journal.*

Imagine my surprise when the article was published (*English Journal,* Vol. 94, No. 4, March 2005); I hadn't believed my writing skills were above adequate. Months later, I was more than shocked to receive an award for the article, probably because few were writing about education and TBI. An Edwin M. Hopkins Award was presented to me in Nashville, TN, at the annual meeting of the National Council of Teachers of English (NCTE) in 2006. This was during my first full-time year of teaching students with learning disabilities. I invited my mother to attend the recognition luncheon and ceremony with me, for she was largely responsible for my recovery and was an English teacher herself.

I admit, reluctantly, that my article was originally filled with venom for the teachers who ignored or avoided me in high school. My guidance counselor, Richard Mock, and a priceless English teacher, Mary Storch, edited out my most brutal complaints. They said my personal whining would detract from the impact of the problems of students with TBI everywhere, so I deleted a great deal of personal bitterness. Soon I was able to Google "Kelly Bouldin and TBI." Having

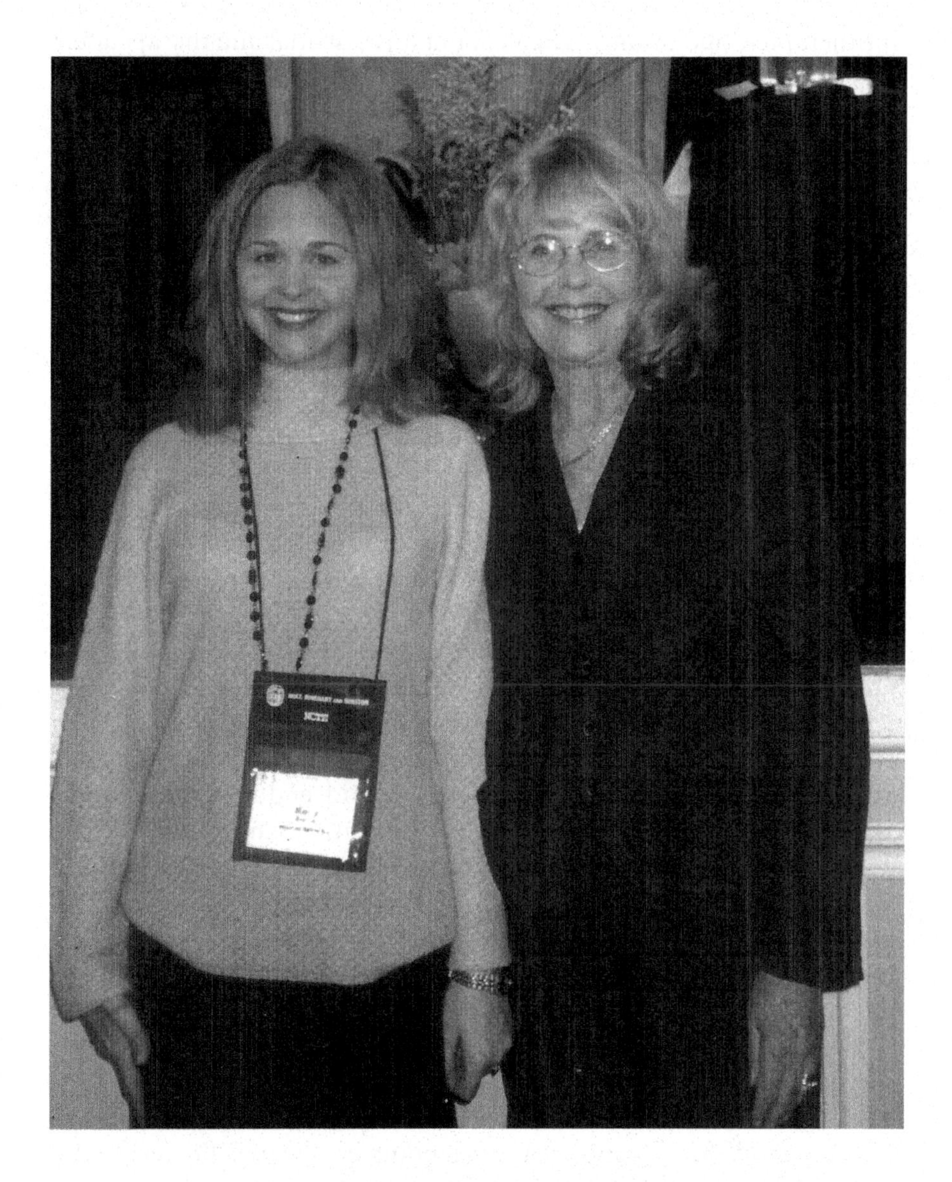

Kelly and her Mother attending the NCTE Conference, 2006

one's own words and feelings published is a true epiphany. I gained the confidence to write my own story, and began the work you are reading now. It is painful and beyond horrible to remember what came before, the therapies, operations, ridicule... but it is essential and therapeutic. I was and am compelled.

I met a speaker at the NCTE luncheon, Alice Sebold, author of *The Lovely Bones*. Her haunting story is now a major film, but her words to me that day filled me with conviction. Sebold asked if I could tell from *Lovely Bones* that she herself had been raped. I said, "No." She went on to recount that while in therapy post-rape, she met numerous families whose daughters had been killed after rape, and whose killers had never been found or convicted. She had been a teenager like me when disaster struck. Sebold said she had begun writing *Lucky*, her own painful memoir, but that the voices of young women who didn't survive their rapists kept interrupting her attempts. She finally put *Lucky* down and wrote *The Lovely Bones*, a story told from the unusual point of view of a dead girl. The voices haunting her were louder than her own voice, and thus Sebold inspired me to write more about TBI, regardless of my temptation to put bad memories behind me.

Another NCTE speaker was delayed that day. Holocaust survivor Elie Wiesel, author of *Night* and activist for human rights, was scheduled to be present, but his plane was delayed. Thinking of reading *Night* in high school, I had another epiphany. I was not the only attendant at the NCTE convention who had endured catastrophe. Wiesel had lost his family in Nazi concentration camps. He had endured the camps, and lived to tell his tale in writing. Creating out of pain may just be essential to full recovery. At any rate, I regret not having heard or met Wiesel. I regret that his foundation lost most of its money in the Bernie Madoff scandal. I regret not shaking the hand of the man who wrote: "I will never forget that night... never."

Perhaps I should also mention that the writing of another Holocaust survivor helped me frequently with TBI symptoms. My cousin George Naff, a counselor, introduced me to the late Viktor Frankl's book *Man's Search for Meaning*. At that point in my life, I'd received a library of so-called "self-help" books, most of which were boring. But Frankl's work was compelling. He called his variant of psychiatry Logotherapy, which reflected that without finding meaning in life, one cannot find happiness. Frankl recommends a technique he calls "paradoxical intention." An example is a patient who cannot sleep, so the doctor recommends trying hard to stay awake all night—and ironically, the patient falls asleep. I tried paradoxical intention often when, for instance, trying not to spill coffee. I would will my hand to shake—and it didn't. I would try to cut meat and throw food off the plate... and it stayed there. I began studying Frankl's book like a Bible. One of his remarks in *Man's Search for Meaning* lingers in my mind... it helps me justify the worst moments of my recovery:

"An abnormal reaction to an abnormal situation is normal behavior."

Frankl also mentions an antidote for mental anguish. He believed humor was one of the "soul's weapons in the fight for self-preservation." I wish I had read Frankl in high school, especially because he emphasizes my favorite Nietzsche quotation:

"Was mich nicht umbringt, macht mich stärker"—"That which does not kill me makes me stronger."

Prior to my experiences in Nashville, I met my husband, who also enjoys the music of *U2*. I met Brad through mutual friends and we immediately hit it off. The two of us were inseparable from that day forward. Brad wasn't familiar with TBI, but he didn't mind the negative side effects associated with the disability. He did, however, feel the occasional pang of frustration with my poor memory, which is totally understandable. I often become frustrated with myself when I forget little, yet important variances in my daily routine. I had a terrible time initially remembering Brad's last name. It wasn't until I asked to see his driver's license photo that I was able to see how Brad's last name was spelled. I was then able to create a mental picture of the name and successfully retain it.

Another added bonus was Brad's obsession with spectator sports. Unable to compete myself, I'd fallen in love with college football and basketball, and with the Boston Celtics. In 2008, Brad and I flew up to Boston to visit my sister, and to see game 6 of the NBA playoffs. The Celtics smashed the Los Angeles Lakers and won their 17th NBA championship. While riding the subway back to our car, Brad looked at me and exclaimed, "This is the best year of my life. I'm 33 years old (Larry Bird's jersey number), I got to see the Boston Celtics win the NBA Championship, and I married my best friend." I remember thinking how lucky I was to have found such a caring man. My next thought was I hoped he knew where we were going and when we needed to exit the subway car... welcome to the thoughts of a TBI survivor! My husband has an excellent sense of direction and easily guided me back to our car that night.

Looking back on previous relationships, I finally realized why, in the midst of graduate school graduation and encroaching adulthood, I was finally capable of sustaining a meaningful romantic relationship. George Santayana wrote the famous quote warning, "Those who cannot learn from history are doomed to repeat it," and this had been my main difficulty. My memory deficits were keeping me from accurately remembering negative occurrences that resulted in the ending of numerous relationships. I wasn't learning from my own history. Thus, I replayed similar dating scenarios repeatedly without observing the seemingly obvious patterns. If I had only kept a "dating diary," highlighting the pluses and minuses of each relationship, I might have been spared some heartache! In many instances, I had chosen to date men with significant problems of their own, those who had also experienced failure and loss. I hadn't exactly "dated down," but sought horizontal relationships which gave me a sense of security... even though it was undoubtedly a false one.

I forgot from one year to the next the scales in life were not balanced as I had hoped—TBI deficits didn't "balance" or "cancel out" alcoholism, or the death of a brother, or something similar. My accident and resulting TBI had stolen my adolescence. I missed the essential trial and error period high school provided for relationship adjustments. When I began evaluating my personal history, I spoke with several family members who said, "You gained self-confidence from your graduate degree and signed teaching contract." Yes, I agreed with these observations.

My self-esteem was buoyed by obtaining these goals, and for the first time post-TBI, I felt ready to be a positive, successful partner. Interestingly, I met my husband, Brad, shortly after gaining my new sense of worth. But growing concerns about my ability to actually teach in a classroom continued to mount; however, Brad was there with me to hold my hand.

And so I began to teach school. In preparation, I wrote my philosophy of education:

> I believe that anyone can learn more than they currently know. Any student who is taught with clarity, creativity, variety, humor, and compassion can exceed his or her expectations, for the most part. My primary interest in becoming an educator is not to teach students who need little assistance. I

want to instruct those who are disabled in some way, as I was and still am. This is why I obtained my certification in K-12 instruction, specializing in children with disabilities. I will always remember the various modifications made for me in high school and college. Without them, I would have been denied the joys of learning new ideas and skills.

Also, I want to help students to grow intellectually while increasing self-esteem. Students who perceive themselves as "different" are already on their way to becoming lost in public education. Their emotions and negative feelings can mask the joy inherent in the learning process.

It has always been important for me to allow students to give me feedback on what they need in the way of academic help. I also want them to feel they can come to me if they have a problem with anything, academic or otherwise. Before venturing into college or the working world, disabled students need to feel comfortable with telling future teachers or employers exactly what they will need—either in the classroom (accommodations and/or modifications) or in the workplace.

I will always assess students fairly, with as much flexibility as necessary. No students of mine will fail unless no effort is made on their parts. I will use portfolios, performances, essays, short answer, etc. to abide by students' accommodations dictated in their IEPs. If a student feels she/he would be more successful with a word bank during a test and I feel the request has merit, I'll provide a word bank.

I will enter the classroom to prepare my students to learn. I see no point in "trick" questions, unless testing for higher order, analytical skills.

I'll do my best not to use methods which are unfair due to the nature of a physical or learning disability. For example, I will give guided tests to students with dyscalculia (a learning disability in math), oral tests for those with dysgraphia (a disability adversely affecting one's handwriting) and TBI in pertinent cases.

I will use computers whenever possible in my classroom, as the disabled do very well when working with assistive technology. As technology develops (like Dragon Speaking Softly), I will incorporate its use when needed.

~ ~ ~

Today I follow the same philosophy. I'm still training my "post-TBI-self" using any information available. I'd love to say my career involves teaching viable strategies to other students with TBI, but it doesn't—sadly.

As my full-time teaching career began, I found no school locally with a need for teachers in this rarified field. The need for a paycheck drives everyone, including me, so I accepted a position in special education. My first position, which I was fortunate to obtain, was teaching in the Johnson Academic Center (JAC) at Forsyth Country Day School (FCDS) near Winston-Salem. The JAC opened in 2001 with the generous donation of Junior and Lisa Johnson. There I worked one-on-one with students who needed support services, and I learned to adapt my skills to each child's individual needs. The resources available at FCDS were tremendous, from the Childress Activities Center (CAC) for exercise, to the JAC for specialized education.

While working with children with varying needs, I discovered the writings of Dr. Edward M. Hallowell. In his book, *CrazyBusy: Overstretched, Overbooked, and About to Snap!* Hallowell writes:

> It is fine to believe that multitasking is a skill necessary in the modern world, but to believe it is an equivalent substitute for single-minded focus on one task is incorrect. You will not be doing any of these tasks as effectively as you would if you were doing them one at a time.

Finally, a man after my own heart! My experiences as a rookie teacher involved learning to multitask, to recall dozens of names, write progress reports, attend staff meetings, shoot off e-mails, actually teach classes, and never forget the needs of students at any given time. Naturally, I forgot a few meetings in my first year, and without benevolent mentors, I might have "crashed and burned" in year one. Hallowell, on the other hand, gave me permission do to things well—one at a time—and to stop worrying about minor errors I made as a new teacher who also wanted to "have a life"—and to publish someday. I no longer believe that multitasking is more than doing a number of things rather badly, which is why I'm strongly against cell phone usage and texting in cars—which can lead to accidents, which can lead to TBI.

Two years later, I accepted a second-grade assistant position at Summit School, where my own education had begun. I finally felt capable of learning an entire classroom of names. I had also followed research on the strong correlation existing between TBI and fatigue. My new position was part-time (supposedly) and would allow me more time to rest, more time to write about head trauma. I felt able to focus entirely on the special needs of my "pull out" groups in the second-grade classroom.

One particular classroom event made me smile at the privilege of teaching children. In the craziness of the day, I was concerned that I might forget about a mandatory parent-teacher open house. I had written the time and place on my arm, just like I had done in high school. Noah looked down at the black markings on my arm and said, "Is that really necessary for a teacher, Mrs. Darmofal?"

"For me it is!" I replied with a smile.

"Oh," said this second-grader. "I think I'd rather just stay clean!"

So would I, Noah, I thought to myself. I'm just doing the best I can with the cards I've been dealt!

15 The TBI Epidemic Rages On

> "To know what is right and not do it is the worst cowardice."
>
> – Confucius

The beauty and simplicity of a student like Noah returns me to the original intent of this memoir, which is to present, through my individual pain, a problem regarding education today. Noah will most likely not suffer from traumatic brain injury, but I believe he is more likely to die from TBI than any other single cause:

- "TBI is the most common cause of death and disability of children in the United States" (Keyser-Marcus et al., 2002).
- "Traumatic brain injuries represent the leading cause of death and disability in young adults in industrialized countries" (Schroeter et al., 2010).
- People with TBI "have an increased risk of death by suicide (3-4 times greater than for the general population)..." (Simpson & Tate, 2007).

Why is the public so unaware? We read every day about NFL players and concussion lawsuits. We know our soldiers are receiving "blast" concussions.

According to the Brain Injury Association of America (2014) www.biausa.org:

- 5.3 million Americans live with a long-term disability as a result of TBI.
- An estimated 2.5 million children and adults in the U.S. sustain a traumatic brain injury (TBI) and another

795,000 individuals sustain an acquired brain injury (ABI) from non-traumatic causes each year.

- The annual cost of TBI to society exceeds *$76.5 billion.*

The CDC (2014) concurs: 2.5 million new TBI's occur yearly; falls are the leading cause of TBI, followed by blunt force trauma, and thirdly, automobile crashes (such as mine).

Perhaps there is confusion in the CDC (2014) category of "injuries", which are reported to cause more U.S. deaths up to age 44 than any other cause. TBI is surely an injury! Statistics are valuable but often misleading. Multiple sources list TBI as the leading cause of young death in America. Those who go back to school must have help!

The research conducted by Glang et al. (2004) is, however, disturbingly clear. This study reveals that as few as 14,456 American public school students are certified "TBI"—yet an estimated 390,000 should be receiving services. TBI is definitely a "high-incidence medical event, [but] it remains a low-incidence disability in the field of special education" (Glang et al., 2004).

A more recent report by Gordon, Oswald, Vaughn, Connors, & Brown (2013) is more shocking:

> TBI is not an orphan disease affecting only 25,000 children... most children with mild TBI will have no long-term challenges triggered by the injury. But the one-in-five children who do have persisting symptoms after a mild brain injury translates to more than one million U.S. schoolchildren (age 5-15) who have experienced a medically treated TBI and are currently symptomatic....[3]

We owe our children more.

[3] "State of the States: Meeting the Educational Needs of Children with Traumatic Brain Injury," www.biausa.org/biaa-position-papers.htm

Happily Ever After?

> "There is no real ending. It's just the place where you stop the story."
>
> – Frank Herbert

I didn't want to conclude my story until I knew how it would end. Of course, the story of TBI is an uphill, never-ending battle. However, I did manage to complete high school, graduate from college, and then graduate school. I didn't perform well at first in the workplace, but after a few failures, I found success with employment that allows me to be useful. My energy and mental capacities are smaller than they were before my TBI, but what I have, I can use as well as anyone.

Will I keep having TBI-related problems? Of course. A blind man rarely sees again, but adapts to the world using other senses more effectively. I am trying to prioritize my goals. My husband deals with, but understands my struggles and failures. For example, we went on a recent trip to the mountains so that I could be a bridesmaid in a friend's wedding. I took care to pack everything I needed: the pearl earrings, the dress, the right shoes, the gift. I forgot to MapQuest the directions for my husband, and we got lost. This is the way my brain works. I can recall all I need within limits, and on this trip, I chose to prioritize the wedding paraphernalia, but I let my husband down. If I had known that I would have to choose whether my memory would retain either the correct jewelry or the vital directions, I would have obviously chosen the directions. This choice would have made my husband much happier as well. However, I'm still learning what is possible for me and what my limitations are. Yes, I still hate myself when I'm not perfect. So I shift my priorities every day. For the next trip, my husband's needs will come first, even if I forget the pearls.

My story is about forgiveness and love, and about three enemies: fear, anxiety, and time. Luckily there are medications for the first two. The final enemy shows itself a little every day, as a person with disability never has enough time to do all the daily chores of life. Time still runs out each day before I accomplish goals, but each year is better than the last. I'm still afraid of failure and afraid of letting others down. I fear abandonment, loss of love, and forgetting minor details that are important to someone else.

My last note of advice to the disabled: "You're good enough, just as you are." These words are, at times, more important than "I love you."

The last challenge for me is to accept myself as I am, for after years of rushing to improve, it's hard to stop. I've also got to stop thinking I'm the only person in the world with problems. I seem to forget that, as patience has never come easily to me.

Forgiveness? For all who rejected me, laughed at me, became angry with my forgetfulness, I want to forgive. After all, forgiveness is an essential part of recovery. I think there are only one or two people left for me to find peace with... and I'm still trying.

Epilogue

Frequently Asked Questions (Kelly)

As an educator I've learned numerous tips for setting up a functional classroom, as well as contemporary strategies and philosophies for educating students. However, as a student I've learned little or nothing concerning the needs of students with TBI. Out of this void, I began writing papers on the subject and will speak publicly, advocating for individuals with TBI in the future. I include frequently asked questions for anyone with an interest.

Why Did You Decide To Publish a Memoir Now?

Please know there are numerous reasons for my mental trip back to the hell of 1992. Clearly, I want the American educational system to train educators to help students with mild, moderate, and severe TBI. Yet another reason for baring my soul is to create awareness to the needs of suffering United States veterans. American soldiers have been returning from Iraq and Afghanistan for years now, and thousands are afflicted with mild, moderate and severe TBI; IAVA or the Iraq Afghanistan Veterans of America (2011) states: "Between 10 and 20 percent of Iraq and Afghanistan vets have suffered a TBI." Most suffer a TBI merely from the blast of nearby explosions; no wound is visible. Others endure multiple wounds including brain injuries. Anyone who reads newspapers and watches television is aware of the story of Bob Woodruff, who received head injuries in 2006 after a roadside bomb exploded near his vehicle; he was then a war correspondent in Iraq. Woodruff's injuries were open-head, and he had several consecutive surgeries. After 37 days in coma, he began a long process of rehabilitation similar to my own. Like me, he chose to continue writing as a means of therapy. Like me, he responds that he is "slower" than he once was. Like me, he may have recovered more quickly by keeping his mind as active and analytical as possible.

Did Other TBI Memoirs Influence You?

Bob Woodruff and his wife Lee have written a wonderful book: *In an Instant: A Family's Journey of Love and Healing*. The need for Lee and Bob Woodruff to co-author a memoir of TBI is similar to my need to work with someone close to me. Memories are dimmed or erased by brain injury, and Woodruff clearly did not wish to wait 22 years as I did. He is a brave man. I could not face my painful memories quite as soon. I feared no one would like me, hire me, love me. Yet Woodruff's Foundation [http://remind.org/] is creating awareness of those like me who are not drastically impaired in the long term. Those with TBI who are mildly or moderately impaired often receive insufficient help and attention—and yet their needs are desperate. Recently, I listened to a radio broadcast discussing ten thousand returning veterans suffering from TBI, who could not qualify for assistance, or had not been correctly diagnosed. Their pain is my pain. I know.

Interestingly, in his memoir Bob Woodruff writes:

> ...there is no exact count of soldiers with traumatic brain injuries.... According to studies done at Walter Reed Army Medical Center in Washington, D.C., 67% of wounded men and women coming out of Iraq... have some degree of head injury. (*In an Instant,* 2008, p. 276.)

The creator of the comic strip *Doonesbury* is also helping greatly to create TBI awareness. I highly recommend Gary Trudeau's *Signature Wound: Rocking TBI*. Trudeau's character Toggle wears an eye patch identical to the one I wore and was embarrassed by (but Toggle doesn't seem embarrassed). His speech is halting like mine was, and he also needs the assistance of his mother and friends as I once did. Toggle finds a true love who accepts him, as I did, but he has to choose between obligations; for him time is also the enemy. Traumatic brain injury is indeed the signature wound of modern veterans, and I applaud Trudeau for his tribute to veterans with traumatic brain injuries.

"You Look Great!": Strategies for Living Inside a Brain Injury, by John C. Byler with Laura Ricard, PhD, is filled with strategies to assist those recovering from TBI in dealing with a "new normal."

Over My Head: A Doctor's Own Story of Head Injury from the Inside Looking Out by Claudia L. Osborn, was the first memoir about surviving TBI that my mother and I read; Osborn comforted us—we felt less alone in the world.

After TBI, What Were Your Worst Problems? Best Solutions?

My worst problems were stress, anxiety, and fear, and my best teachers were calm and made me feel at ease in their classrooms. I suffered from an extreme case of culture shock. After being an elite student treated with respect, I was treated like an idiot and rarely allowed privileges, like going to the bathroom alone. I also felt abandoned. I'm still dealing with this issue.

Another huge problem is flooding. A flood is the overwhelming feeling often associated with tremendous stress. When any person, but especially someone with TBI, experiences a flood, the mind goes completely blank and the body may shake uncontrollably. In a flood I couldn't remember my name, much less answers to my teachers' questions.

What Helped You the First Year in School?

What helped me the most in academia was having a very specific IEP. Emotionally I was helped by common courtesies. I recommend that teachers treat students with TBI normally, avoiding condescension. Those with TBI don't want to seem different.

What Symptoms were Most Evident as a TBI Student in Public School?

My worst problems in school included an auditory processing disorder, anterograde and retrograde amnesia, receptive and expressive aphasia, monotone speech that was slow and, at times, a bit slurred, a bilateral hand impairment resulting in the shaking of the right side of my body, and an irregular gait due to muscle trauma and double vision (diplopia) .

Since TBI Documentation was New to Your School, How Did You Cope?

I used numerous strategies when I felt overwhelmed by my disabilities. I would close my eyes and think of a peaceful place, like the beach, or simply zone out for a moment or two. I could divide my workload into manageable segments, and then attack it one assignment at a time.

Doing something completely unrelated, like going to the gym or walking. I would try to make fun of the situation, or find something unrelated to laugh about.

Cleaning something always helped, giving me visible satisfaction. Occasionally I would call a close friend and whine.

Music and singing (even though I'm tone-deaf) often lightened my mood.

What are some specific classroom strategies?

Assume nothing

The student may not know what he or she once knew, or what has been forgotten.

This was definitely true for me. When I first returned to high school and sat down in class, I was asked to take notes on the day's lecture. When I got home later that day, the notes I took so carefully were horribly jumbled together. At first my mother simply thought that I'd been doodling. She was perturbed.

That day in class I had taken notes with each line on top of another line, beginning in the center of the page. No one said notes should be taken at the beginning of a line—or from left to right. There are countless obstacles facing a person with a TBI. Yet all my mother had to do *was remind me* of correct sequencing; my notes improved.

Keep a sense of humor with students recovering from TBI

A sense of humor should be maintained with a student exhibiting socially inappropriate behavior. I had choice words with the administration when I came back to school, but I was just trying to be friendly. With luck and patience, the odd behaviors will decrease. (Luckily, I didn't cuss as much as other patients I know in the TBI recovery stage.)

Use cues or "triggers"

"Triggers" for testing may be a necessity for the student with TBI to remember an intended response. The letter "L", for instance, could help me recall "Lincoln."

Don't demand handwriting unless appropriate

Allow those with TBI to listen in class, use laptops or other assistive devices....or—

Provide note takers

In the '90s some teachers still used carbon paper instead of copying machines... times have changed.

Prepare Word Banks for cueing

I finally had "word banks" added to my IEP. From a list of all state capitals, I could then find Richmond as the capital of Virginia.

Use mnemonic strategies and mind games

They helped me greatly in remembering new material. In my American history class, I needed to remember the names of the five Great Lakes (Superior, Ontario, Michigan, Erie, and Huron). My mother and I came up with S.ome M.en E.at H.airy O.tters to help me remember, and it worked. This kind of strategy tends to be more effective if the phrase is either humorous, personal, or both.

Give extended time when needed

Always allow those with TBI extra time when necessary to complete tests or assignments. Society places too high a premium on speed, which creates stress.

Allow retesting and/or rewriting

Inform students that if they do their best and keep trying, they cannot fail. This will work and decrease flooding.

Never postpone a test for the traumatically brain injured

The simple act of memorizing something new is hard enough. It's simply cruel to reschedule a test on a subject a student has already studied for. The knowledge will probably be lost overnight, and will have to be relearned.

For example, John knows he can remember data for about three days, so he studies all weekend for a test on Monday. The teacher on Monday announces that the test is postponed until Thursday. John must restudy and relearn the same material over again. The same issue concerns completing tests not finished in class. Teachers should give make-up work as soon as possible.

Give wait time

When asking a student with TBI a question, be sure to give plenty of wait time. Processing data is slow for the traumatically brain injured, but answers can come with ample time.

Study the nature of amnesia (anterograde, retrograde)

Amnesia is nothing like the soap operas when characters awaken, fully healthy, but do not know their family. Amnesia is selective; even the student with TBI may not know what has been forgotten. For instance, I recalled the Pythagorean theorem, but had to relearn how to multiply; this took a half hour only. I remembered Shakespeare, but not Judas Iscariot. Teachers mustn't assume knowledge, yet should prepare for students with TBI to have vast knowledge of certain subjects. Their entire memory banks will not have been erased. I, for instance, was totally comfortable on my computer, with all the software.

Never condescend

When students with TBI begin to recover, they may have difficulty recalling what they did an hour ago. This time-limited recall can expand with healing until the student can easily recall what was once forgotten.

If a teacher showed me respect, I was at ease and could respond rather easily to questions. On the other hand, when teachers assumed that I was deficient and used a condescending tone, I would flood. My flooding would thus confirm their uninformed diagnosis of irreparable impairment.

Help the transition from concrete to analytical

Students with TBI may have great difficulty with analytical thought. The first weeks out of coma, my world appeared very literal and concrete. If a friend said, "That girl is hot," I thought she was sweating. Poetry and figures of speech can help this transition. My brain was still swollen, unready for humor and ambiguous speech.

Recognize the student's strengths

The student convalescing from TBI has enough difficulty with memory. He/she definitely doesn't need to be given fill-in-the blank tests with no word bank. Simply seeing empty blanks immediately gave me anxiety attacks, but I could make 100 with the word bank... so I knew the material well.

Use repetition with TBI students

The number of repeats will hopefully decline with time.

Write down all assignments and provide home/cell phone numbers and e-mail addresses

When (not if) the student with TBI loses the paper you've written the homework assignment on, you can provide it again... and again.

Avoid trick questions

When testing, trick questions may confuse those with TBI, and make them answer incorrectly. Life is hard enough with a disability. Don't ask nebulous or confusing questions.

Offer social skills training

This may be essential for students with TBI.

Offer frequent rest breaks

The victim of TBI tires easily and may suffer *extreme fatigue*.

~ ~ ~

I believe that for many years, students in American schools with severe TBI either never returned to schools or were placed inappropriately in special education or LD classrooms. Fortunately, TBI certification/classification now exists; the school population of students with TBI is growing, possibly due to improved health care methodology.

Unfortunately, few teachers have had training and experience with TBI, as the classification was added as a separate category of disability to IDEA (Individuals with Disabilities Act) in 1990; autism was added at the same time and receives more attention educationally than TBI, a significant public health problem that is often mistaken for an "orphan disease" that affects few people.

Interestingly, some people feel that students with TBI are similar to LD (learning disabled) students and can be treated in the same fashion. Similarities do exist, but great differences exist as well. The child with TBI must be recognized by each teacher as a separate and different student, and teachers require more education to help such a child.

It is very possible that students with TBI who find their way back to public schools were once gifted students. Think about it: IQ usually diminishes after a severe open- or closed-head injury. If the students are still bright enough to return to school, they may have had quite high IQs before their head traumas.

Doctors may recommend that students recovering from TBI return to their normal school environments as quickly as possible, mainly because these students often suffer amnesia. However, their memories can quickly be triggered back in familiar settings. The reality is, sadly, that students with TBI often return to school before they are cognitively or physically healed. They often seem confused (they are, not recalling names of teachers or locations of classes) and may walk with a limp. They may have speech, vision, and hearing problems, as the brain controls such functions. In other words, such a student may seem unhealthy, clumsy, and out of place in the school environment. However, this is the environment that has the best hopes of healing such a child.

The classroom teacher needs to realize that the student who comes to them with TBI can indeed change and progress rapidly. Improvements for those with TBI often come in spurts, and are sometimes rapid. Or, a student may "plateau" for a time, or move forward and backward. Regression can occur, yet can be caused by stress as well as health issues.

In other words, the teacher doesn't really know what child they will see each day. It might be the slow student today, and the quick student tomorrow—or the scared one. This is a primary difference between the student with LD and the child with TBI; the latter changes each day; the former's symptoms are generally more static (my opinion).

The public school child with TBI has essentially become LD or worse, virtually overnight. Emotional adjustments have to be made. I returned to high school in Winston-Salem, North Carolina following a severe closed-head injury. My IQ was 70 and is now almost double that.... Having suffered memory loss and physical impairments, I needed to know of just one person in the school to turn to when I needed help. Unfortunately, I didn't have *one*. I was alternately sent to guidance, special education teachers, the principal, etc., for my needs. This was different at Salem College, where one professor was my resource teacher and helper. Having one person to help gave me calm and stability.

Sadly, children with TBI may have trouble forming peer groups as they have most likely lost any tact they once possessed. A child with learning differences is not a peer. The child with TBI probably feels smart, but cannot communicate effectively in any fashion for several months. Thus, the appropriate placement is most likely the regular classroom, as strange as that may seem. This child recovering from TBI may belong there in time as memories will likely return. Thus the teacher must realize that rapid improvement is possible with patience, extra time for speaking, questioning and testing, and with compassion.

Also, the student with TBI is probably the best person to consult about modifications during any IEP meeting.

A computer is the friend of students with TBI. It corrects spelling and is very patient. I personally never forgot computer knowledge, but others may.

A computer keyboard is also easier for people with dysgraphia, or poor handwriting, to operate. Do not assume that students with TBI are lazy when they are just slow or confused. Answer questions with patience. Make appropriate accommodations even if they are not included in the IEP.

One wonders if students with TBI who can memorize only for short times, can file these memories for longer periods. I'm not a doctor, but I've recalled lost data from high school, at times, years into the future. I think the memories were filed long-term, but simply couldn't be retrieved at particular moments. I tended to have better recall when units were broken into smaller sections, as tests on one chapter at a time as opposed to tests on four chapters. I'm sure I did my best work when using a multi-sensory approach, reading, writing, speaking, and using my kinesthetic sense.

The iPhone and iPad (along with other handheld, electronic devices) are assets to the student with TBI. Many of the applications, or "apps," which can be added to a person's iPhone or iPad, are either free of charge or can be purchased for a minimal fee. These apps can record classroom lectures with clarity while suppressing background noise, and amplify the voice of a teacher for brain-injured students with auditory disabilities. Another popular app combines voice recording with a transcription service, allowing a lecture to be recorded and automatically converted into writing. The Pic-Z Tag application for the iPhone allows a student with expressive difficulties to innovatively introduce himself/herself to fellow classmates without speaking. The iPhone converts into an electronic nametag, which would have assisted someone like me who had expressive aphasia coupled with slurred speech.

As with learning disabilities, the severity of problems will vary with TBI convalescents. Symptoms will differ according to which part of the brain was damaged. However, fast and remarkable progress is possible for the young because their brains are still growing. This is the good news. The bad news is that TBI is on the rise in America and our educational system must attend.

It is hard for me to believe that people are still unfamiliar with the acronym TBI, despite its growing prevalence in today's society.

"Every 23 seconds someone in the U.S. sustains a Traumatic Brain Injury"; (It could happen to you... today. The Brain Injury Association of North Carolina/BIANC, ncbraininjury.net.).

Some victims will die, but many will live and be disabled forever. It could easily happen to you. Do you know how to prevent a traumatic brain injury? Do you know what to do if someone you love acquires a TBI?

The following statistics should motivate you to learn more about and take steps toward preventing a traumatic brain injury for yourself or those you love. According to Mason, M.P. (2014), Brainline.org:

- If you were to experience a severe brain injury today, it would cost anywhere from $60,000 to $1.8 million dollars to care for you over your lifetime.
- The age groups at highest risk for TBI are 0 to 4 year olds, 15 to 19 year olds, and adults aged 65 and older.
- African Americans have the highest death rate from TBI.
- Males are approximately 1.5 times as likely as females to sustain a TBI.

Some sources list a higher cost in dollars. BIANC, based on 2014 data from the CDC, states: "The average lifetime cost for caring for a person with brain injury now exceeds $4 million."

The BIAA, BIANC, and the CDC provide fact sheets (see www.ImLostInMyMind for links) with fluctuating data from 2003 to 2014—and the facts are astounding.

In my home State of North Carolina:

- Brain injury is the leading cause of death and disability among young people in our State (BIANC, 2014).
- TBI strikes seventy-five families each week [just] in North Carolina (BIANC, 2014).
- According to CDC data in 2007, 65,989 people in North Carolina were seen in emergency departments for traumatic brain injury and 4,000 will acquire lifelong disabilities.

Across America, the TBI epidemic is raging. According to authorities:

- TBI is a major public health issue and cause of death and disability in children and adults. It occurs 8 times more often than the number of people annually diagnosed with breast cancer and 34 times more often than the number of new cases of HIV/AIDS (BIANC, 2003).

- More people will sustain a brain injury each year, than are diagnosed with breast cancer, HIV, AIDS, multiple sclerosis (MS), and spinal cord injuries combined (BIANC, 2014).
- Over 1,365,000 people annually are treated in an Emergency Department for TBI (CDC, 2014).
- 52,000 people will die yearly of TBI (BIAA, 2014).
- 275,000 people will be hospitalized due to TBI (BIAA, 2014).
- About 75% of TBIs that occur each year are concussions or other forms of mild traumatic brain injury (MTBI) (BIAA, 2014).
- According to "Brain Injury in Children", BIAA, 2014) Traumatic brain injury (TBI) is the leading cause of disability and death in children and adolescents in the U.S. According to the CDC, the two age groups at greatest risk for TBI are age 0-4 and 15-19. Among those aged 0 to 19, each year an average of:
- 62,000 children sustain brain injuries requiring hospitalization as a result of motor vehicle crashes, falls, sports injuries, physical abuse, and other causes
- 564,000 children are seen in hospital emergency departments for TBI and released.
- Experts believe well over 1 million children in America acquire a TBI each year (Gordon, Oswald, Vaughn, Connors, & Brown, 2013).

As stated earlier:

- Traumatic Brain Injuries are the leading cause of death of American children (Keyser-Marcus et al., 2002).

What Can People Do to Help?

There are numerous measures that can be taken to prevent traumatic brain or head injuries. For instance, people can choose to obey seat belt laws, which would prevent a sudden blow to the head against the dashboard or the side of the car.

Wearing protective head gear, such as helmets, when riding horses, bicycling, or engaging in contact sports (even field hockey players, who do not always require helmets, need head protection from the severe blow of a hockey stick) would also help. However, there have been recent reports that negate the safety of some helmets due to the lack of helmet regulations. Be an informed buyer.

Be careful when skiing near trees, as skiing is another cause of head injury. Again, head protection can be worn.

Make sure you carry enough liability insurance. Special policies can protect a family from the under-insured or uninsured motorist. Most people do not carry enough insurance to cover the costs of TBI. At minimum, a one million dollar policy is needed which can cost as little as $200 annually.

Protect the very young and the very old from unnecessary falls. Guardrails, gates, and other measures can save someone from acquiring a TBI.

Drive defensively at all times. Don't text, talk, or drink while driving.

Be kind.

~ ~ ~

Follow Kelly's website at www.imlostinmymind.com for helpful URLs and other information related to TBI.

Where are they now? (people mentioned in the text)

For those who have interest in individuals mentioned earlier:

- Dr. Amanda Waugh Moy is now working as an ER physician in California, having earned a full scholarship to medical school at the University of North Carolina-Chapel Hill. My husband and I danced at her wedding to the hilarious Dr. Ron in the Virgin Islands. We talk and text daily.
- Lee did find a "normal girl" to love and is now happily married and the father of beautiful children.
- Cousin Emily didn't keep the ring or the "guy." She soon married a wonderful man and is the mother of two adorable daughters.
- Amanda "Gardner" Porter married a professor of music and sings professionally.
- Mitzy, (Mitzy's) Buddie, and Macy keep me both sane and happy.
- Tyler is still my role model, happily married with two daughters who love their Aunt Kelly no matter what.
- Zach is married, and invited me to his wedding. He is doing well and has an adorable son.
- Chad, the noisy passenger, took me out once in '93 and left me at a baseball game.
- Marc still gives me the Vulcan salute.
- LaLa still comes whenever I need her, minus the raincoat.
- Carolyn Bouldin is an academic coach (sometimes homebound) for victims of TBI and other disabilities.
- My father is happy I'm finally an excellent driver.

Frequently Asked Questions (Kelly's Mom)

Have You Found Any Colleges Training Teachers of Students With TBI?

During our last online search, Kelly and I located Coastline Community College in California which offers one class, and one program at the University of Central Florida. My librarian sister discovered the latter recently, and her "search" abilities are enormous. I found one more—if one happens to live in England, there is a class at the Worcester College of Technology. Please contact Kelly's publisher if you know of others.

What New Developments Interest You in TBI Research?

The "checklight" developed by Reebok and MC10! This skullcap can measure impact to the brain; if the light goes on, athletes can be removed from play.

Also, research by the Virginia Tech and Wake Forest University School of Bioengineering and Sciences: their STAR system (Summation of Tests for the Analysis of Risk) is evaluating football helmets which can alert coaches to remove athletes from games; concussions are the most common sports injury in many sports. A pilot study at Reagan High School involving such helmets in Winston-Salem encourages us; students with TBI are a sad reality.

Recently the *Winston-Salem Journal* (2013) noted: the NCAA donated $399,999 to the Matthew Gfeller Sports-Related TBI Research Center at UNC-CH and the University of Wisconsin; more must be learned about the effects of concussions on athletes now and in the future. In 2011 in North Carolina the Gfeller-Waller Concussion Awareness Act was signed into law; this legislation requires schools to have an emergency action plan in effect for injured athletes—as well as a safety training program and a protocol for allowing athletes to be cleared prior to return to play. Kelly's memoir pays tribute to Matt Gfeller and the efforts of his family regarding TBI and sports.

However, Kelly and I are more involved with the "black hole" in the education of students with TBI. Over a million school children with TBI are not receiving the help they need (Gordon, Oswald, Vaughn, Connors, & Brown, 2013). Another study (2008) at the University of Dayton (Gfroerer et al.) agrees with our view that teacher training is woefully inadequate. Please read a report by Glang et al. (2004) that suggests an inexpensive way for school systems to train their teachers in helping TBI-certified students, via statewide consulting teams. Also note that TBI training generally comes under the special education umbrella—which is inadequate. Hux et al. (2013) emphasizes the need for colleges and universities to increase focus on emerging TBI school populations, stating that "Improving academic preparation for special educators regarding TBI is imperative for effectively identifying, assessing, and serving student survivors."

Where Does The Layman Turn for Help? Or the Teacher with Interest in TBI?

Since the Internet became available, Kelly and I have followed the websites of Brain Injury Association of America (BIAA) and (Brain Injury Association of North Carolina (BIANC). From Kelly's correspondence with the BIAA we have learned that:

- There is a program called the Academy of Certified Brain Injury Specialists (ACBIS) to certify professionals providing services to those with TBI; some (but not all) are educators... hopefully their number is growing. Also, webinars and print materials are available via the BIAA. See: www.acbis.pro/. In our home State of North Carolina, we recommend http://bianc.net/resources/education_and_training/CBIS/index.html
- Some states are ahead of others in addressing TBI educational needs: See the excellent tutorials from New York at http://www.projectlearnet.org/index.html; also BrainSTEPS (kudos to Pennsylvania) with a focus on educational re-entry.

Still we pray that teacher training in colleges and universities will pick up this torch and run. As this memoir goes into print, BIAA notes there are currently 266 educators nationwide certified as Brain Injury Specialists by the Academy of Certified Brain Injury Specialists. Over 10% are from Pennsylvania (due to their BrainSTEPS program). Progress for students with TBI in education is slow... but it is progress. Educators, take note!

Appendix: Study Guide and Activities

1. Poetry is surely a motif in Kelly's memoir of TBI. *Why was poetry important to Kelly?*
2. In which portions of the memoir does humor emerge as an important coping device? *Discuss.*
3. Diaries and other epistolary writings have often provided unique insights in literature. *In your opinion, was Kelly's mother Carolyn wise to record Kelly's painful convalescence that she gave to her years later? Or are some painful memories best left forgotten?*
4. Kelly mentions that she experienced "culture shock" in school post-TBI. Once an honors student, she believed teachers treated her, as a disabled student, differently and with less respect. *Do you feel her judgment is a fair one, and have you seen or experienced a similar situation?*
5. Would you agree/disagree with Kelly that friends in "low places" can be more important than friends in high places?
6. Kelly cites other "survivor stories" as important to her convalescence—particularly victims of the Holocaust. Do you agree with Victor Frankl's remark, *"An abnormal reaction to an abnormal situation is normal behavior"?* Give an example(s) from personal experience.
7. Several metaphors define Kelly Bouldin Darmofal and her mother. *Why is her mother a "shovel" and why did Kelly decline to be a "cobra"?*
8. Isolation (or abandonment) is a theme in this memoir; *do "hope and optimism" emerge as more important themes – or not?* Another theme of this memoir is the problems inherent in large

bureaucracies; *why does Kelly take pains to describe the various positive things teachers did to help her? Can you list a few?*

9. What lessons can caretakers learn from Kelly's memoir? Teachers? Survivors? *Make lists.*
10. Dr. Frank B. Wood[4] says of Kelly, "She understands mediocrity as the great millstone around the neck of education." *Divide into small groups and elaborate. Also: consider why Dr. Wood calls Kelly's memoir "revolutionary."*
11. Britt Armfield, in a letter, shared a favorite Bible quote with the Bouldins: "I consider that our present sufferings are not worth comparing with the glory that will be revealed in us." – ROMANS 8:18. *Relate this passage to Kelly's real and spiritual journey.*
12. Consider Kelly's view that her male friends were more reliable than most female friends. *From personal experience, why might this be so, or not?*
13. Kelly Darmofal hopes to explode some of the myths about TBI, including: 1) the assumption that life post-TBI cannot have a happy ending entailing a reasonably full recovery; and 2) that one's personality post-TBI is permanently altered in all cases. That said, what were three manifestations of her early personality changes? *Which were physical? Which may have been caused by outside influences?*
14. Kelly's relationships naturally did change after her TBI. *How did social activities enhance her recovery?*

Vocabulary to consider:

Anterograde amnesia
Bilateral hand impairment
Diplopia
Expressive aphasia
Glasgow Coma Scale
Perseverance/perseveration
Posturing
Purposeful motion/movement
Retrograde amnesia
Socially inappropriate or unacceptable behavior

---

[4] Frank Wood is professor emeritus of neurology/neuropsychology at Wake Forest School of Medicine, an international expert on Dyslexia, and an ordained Baptist minister.

Further Topics for Research and Class Discussion:

- What is the role of family in recovery from TBI?
- Do caretakers need their own caretakers?
- Does travel and "time away from family" play a part in recovering from TBI?
- Locate/discuss: The Individuals with Disabilities Act and the Americans with Disabilities Act

TBI Workshop I:

- Handicap the class.
- Pass out eye patches to be worn by participants (or use safety glasses smeared with Vaseline).
- Pass out mittens to be worn on each person's dominant hand.
- Pass out earplugs to some students to mute hearing.
- Give flashcards to each person; each card lists a different handicap.
- (one card reads: YOU MAY NOT SPEAK, another reads: WAIT 30 SECONDS BEFORE ANSWERING ORAL QUESTIONS, etc.)
- Teach a poem at rapid speed, possibly by Keats, such as "Ode to a Nightingale"; test immediately with no multiple choices, word banks, or visual clues.
- Allow each person to remove one or more handicaps; retest.
- Discuss why Keats was "half in love with easeful death."
- Allow each person to remove one or more handicaps; retest.
- Conclude with discussion of how healing influences the academic performance of students with TBI over time.

TBI Workshop II:

Hand out copies of IDEA (Individuals with Disabilities Education Act). Work in small groups to relate the law to Kelly's memoir. A second class could relate the ADA (Americans with Disabilities Act) to Kelly and other TBI survivors in the working world.

Acknowledgements

Editorial assistance:

Karen Ackerson, founder and Executive Director of The Writers' Workshop of Asheville, NC and senior editor of the Renbourne Literary Agency

Justin Brewster

Clara G. Fountain

Marc Fountain, technical assistance/photography

I want to give special thanks to those who visited me during the 31 days at Brenner's (forgive me if you didn't sign and I can't remember):

Nathan Beckerman
Tyler Bouldin
Justin Brewster
Kody Brown
Ellon Butler
Glenn Butler
Jacob Chapman
Jeff and Katie Chapell
Anna and Holt Chetwood
Sara Crowder
Ann Brown Crowder
Peter and Lee Culp
Charles Davis
Jack and Lucy Davis
Julia Davis
Myrtie Moon Davis
Suzanne Davis, Derrick, and Ann
Stan and Kirk Elrod
Jimmy Eskridge
Katherine Edwards
Andy Martin
Betty Martin
Charlie Mickey
Courtney Midget
Steve and Margaret Mills
Caroline Mitchell, Nick, "Big C"
Lynda Morris
Jonathan Murphy
Grant Oates
Carey Parker
Chad Parker
Mrs. Norman (Parker)
Jennifer Parks and her mother
Hannah Parrish
Alex Paschold
Annie and Buff Perry
Zach, George, and Patsy Perryman
Holly Pfeffer
Silva Pfefferkorn
Sara Plonk

Butter and Romey Fisher
Meb Faber
John Fagg
Susan Fisher
Nicole Flowers
Mark and Elise Giordano
Raleigh Gregory
Ginger Groce
Lehoma Goode
David Holden
Melanie Johnson
Ann Kenan
Patricia Kenan-Herrman
Aly Kleinmeyer
Kelly and Ashley Knight
Mariah Kulp
Laney (other Young Life leaders)
Aubrey Linville
Nancy Lynn Lockman
Whitney Long
Nicole, Barbara, and Bobby Price
"Ace" Pryor
Jamie Rabb
Emily Reagan
Elizabeth Redden
Michael Rogers and mother
Caroline and Dolores Sanders
Dr. Bob Sawyer
Mike Simone
Judy and Graham Smith
Anna Spaugh
Tasha Thrift
Lindsay Truluck
Dr. Charles Turner
Paige Wagner
Drew Walker
Jessica Wetherhold
Annette Wilson
Diane Wilson
J.D. Wright

And my other guardian angels:

- Dena and Will Anderson
- Joe Powell
- Richard Smiley's "family" on Avalon Rd., the Porters, et al.
- Blake Battaglia
- Rosemary Cerato
- Donna and Herman Darmofal
- Evelyn, Earle, Scottie and Earle III Garrett
- Dr. Frank B. Wood
- The staffs of Camp Thunderbird and Young Life of America/ Winston-Salem
- R.J. Reynolds High School faculty—and
- Mr. Elrod who allowed me to return
- Anne Owen of Peace College
- Salem College faculty and The Class of 2000
- Becky Brown
- Bain Storch and family

- Tricia Smith
- Lara Hanes and family
- Vaughan Penn and family
- Ed, Cece, Edwin, William Bouldin
- Kelton Cofer for sitting and talking with me at a bonfire
- Lois and Gene Raymer and family
- Meredith, Jane, and David Ahles
- Janice Blackburn
- Aisha Dew
- Dr. Sandra Adams
- Dr. David Kelly and his secretary, who always put my modification requests on top of his incoming mail
- Dr. James D. Mattox
- Dr. Grey Weaver
- Louann Reid, former editor of *English Journal*
- Amanda and Ron Moy
- All my "other mothers" (Prissy, Ann, Barbara…you know who you are)
- Volvo – for a safe car with overhead airbags
- My profound thanks to everyone who tried to help me post-9/17/92, but I was too "broken" to understand and remember. Kody, thank you for the '92 Homecoming carnation.
- Thank you to Salem College for allowing me to use their photograph of Oprah Winfrey speaking at the 2000 commencement ceremony.
- Many thanks to the members of Home Moravian Church, the Junior League of Winston-Salem, and the Dogwood Garden Club, who fed my family while I was in coma and awakening!
- Thank you to Summit School – Dr. Ebeling and all staff
- Thank you to Forsyth Country Day School.
- Thank you to the late June Lyday Orton, a former neighbor, and inspiration for always trying another way.
- Thank you to Susan H. Connors, President/CEO/BIAUSA and Greg Ayotte, CBIS, Director of Consumer Services, BIAA
- WFU/BMC and Brenner Children's Hospital – I thank all who saved my life!

~~~

By the time this memoir is published, the incidence of TBI will have greatly increased. Statistics herein will be higher. If you know someone with TBI, please be kind to them and never lose sight of what he or she may, in time, become. *Never give up!*
~~~

Resources

Bibliography of Influential Books

Angelou, Maya. *I Know Why the Caged Bird Sings.* 1969 (autobiography). Ballantine Books; Reissue edition (April 21, 2009). ISBN-10: 0345514408.

Byler, John C. and Ricard, Laura Ph.D. *"You Look Great!": Strategies for Living Inside a Brain Injury* (July 26, 2011). ISBN-13: 978-1463621247.

Conroy, Pat. *The Water is Wide: A Memoir.* 1972. Dial Press Trade Paperback; Reprint edition (March 26, 2002).ISBN-10: 1400008948.

Dickenson, Emily. *The Complete Poems of Emily Dickinson.* Boston, Mass.: Little, Brown, 1960. ISBN: 0316184144; 9780316184144; 0316184136; 9780316184137; National Library: 000933299 LCCN: 60-11646.

Frankl, Viktor. *Man's Search for Meaning.* 1946. New York : Pocket Books, 1963. ISBN: 0671433822; 9780671433826; 0671454625 (pbk.); 9780671454623.

Giffords, Gabrielle and Mark. *Gabby: A Story of Courage, Love and Resilience.* Scribner; Reprint edition (October 9, 2012). ISBN-10: 9781451661071.

Hallowell, Edward M., *CrazyBusy: Overstretched, Overbooked, and About to Snap! Strategies for Handling Your Fast-Paced Life.* Ballantine Books: Reprint edition (March 27, 2007). ISBN-10: 0345482441.

Hillenbrand, Laura. *Unbroken: A World War II Story of Survival, Resilience, and Redemption.* Random House; 1st edition (November 16, 2010). ISBN-10: 1400064163.

Hughes, Langston. *The Collected Works of Langston Hughes.* New York: G. Braziller, 1958. ISBN-13: 9780807600573.

Levine, Mel. *A Mind at a Time.* Simon & Schuster (December 31, 2002). ISBN-10: 0743202236.

Millay, Edna St. Vincent. *Collected Poems of Edna St. Vincent Millay.* Harper Perennial (July 10, 1981). ISBN-10: 0060908890.

Orton, June L. *A Guide to Teaching Phonics.* Educators Publishing Service, Inc; 2nd edition (1975). ISBN-10: 0838802419.

Osborn, Claudia L. *Over My Head: A Doctor's Own Story of Head Injury from the Inside Looking Out.* Kansas City, Andrews McMeel Publishing, 1999. ISBN 0-83625419-8.

Plato. *"The Allegory of the Cave."* In: *The Norton reader; an anthology of Expository prose.* 1969 Rev. English Book xxvii, 1505 p. 22 cm. New York, Norton.

Trudeau, Gary. *Signature Wound: Rocking TBI.* Andrews McMeel Publishing; 1 edition (May 11, 2010). ISBN-10: 0740791966.

Tucker, Bethanie *Tucker Signing Strategies for Reading.* aha! Process, Inc.; Revised edition (January 1, 2001). ISBN-10: 1934583677.

Weisel, Elie. *Night.* New York, NY : Hill and Wang, a division of Farrar, Straus and Giroux, 2006. ISBN: 9780809073566 (hardcover : alk. paper)

Wilson, Barbara. *Wilson Reading System. Parkton, Md.* : York Press, 1988. ISBN: 9780912752143 (pbk.); 0912752157; 9780912752150 LCCN: 88-50703.

Woodruff, Bob and Lee. *In an Instant: A Family's Journey of Love and Healing.* Random House Trade Paperbacks; Reprint edition (February 12, 2008). ISBN-10: 0812978250.

Recommended Readings

in reverse chronological order:

Gordon, W. A., Oswald, J. M., Vaughn, S. L., Connors, S. H., & Brown, M. (2013). *State of the states: Meeting the educational needs of children with traumatic brain injury*. BIAA.

Hux, K., Bush, E., Evans, K., & Simanek, G. (2013). Misconceptions about traumatic brain injury among students preparing to be special education professionals. *Support For Learning*, *28*(3), 109-114. doi:10.1111/1467-9604.12028

Coronado, V. G., McGuire, L. C., Sarmiento, K., Bell, J., Lionbarger, M. R., Jones, C. D., & ... Xu, L. (2012). Trends in Traumatic Brain Injury in the U.S. and the public health response: 1995–2009. *Journal Of Safety Research*, *43*(4), 299-307. doi:10.1016/j.jsr.2012.08.011.

Coronado, V. G., Likang, X., Basavaraju, S. V., McGuire, L. C., Wald, M. M., Faul, M. D., & ... Hemphill, J. (2011). Surveillance for Traumatic Brain Injury-Related Deaths -- United States, 1997-2007. *MMWR Surveillance Summaries*, *60*(SS-5), 1-32.

Schroeter, M.L., Ettrich, B., Menz, M., & Zysset, S. (2010). Traumatic brain injury affects the frontomedian cortex--an event-related fMRI study on evaluative judgments. *Neuropsychologia 48*(1), 185-193.

Glang, A. & Todis, B. (2008). Redefining success: Results of a qualitative study of post-secondary transition outcomes for youth with traumatic brain injury. *Journal of Head Trauma Rehabilitation, 23* (4), 252-263.

Gfroerer, S., Wade, S. L., & Wu, M. (2008). Parent perceptions of school-based support for students with traumatic brain injuries. *Brain Injury*, *22*(9), 649-656. doi:10.1080/02699050802227162

Simpson, G., & Tate, R. (2007). Suicidality in people surviving a traumatic brain injury: Prevalence, risk factors and implications for clinical management. *Brain Injury*, *21*(13/14), 1335-1351. doi:10.1080/02699050701785542.

Bouldin, K. V. (Mar 2005). "TBI: Our teachers are not prepared." *English Journal*, *94* (4), 52.

Glang, A., Tyler, J., Pearson, S., Todis, B., & Morvant, M. (2004). Improving educational services for students with TBI through statewide consulting teams. *Neurorehabilitation*, *19*(3), 219-231.

Keyser-Marcus, L., Briel, L., Sherron-Targett, P., Yasuda, S., Johnson, S., & Wehman, P. (2002). Enhancing the Schooling of Students with Traumatic Brain Injury. *Teaching Exceptional Children*, *34*(4), 62.

Index

CPSIA information can be obtained
at www.ICGtesting.com
Printed in the USA
LVOW01s1654240417
531983LV00003B/210/P